Effective Medical Testifying

Effective Medical Testifying
A Handbook for Physicians

William T. Tsushima, Ph.D.
Clinical Psychologist, Straub Clinic and Hospital, Honolulu

Kenneth K. Nakano, M.D., M.P.H., S.M., F.R.C.P.(C)
Neurologist, Neurological Consultations and Evaluations, Straub Clinic and Hospital, Honolulu

Butterworth–Heinemann

Boston•Oxford•Johannesburg•Melbourne•New Delhi•Singapore

Library of Congress Cataloging-in-Publication Data

Tsushima, William T.
  Effective medical testifying : a handbook for physicians / William T.
Tsushima, Kenneth K. Nakano.
      p.   cm.
  Includes bibliographical references and index.
  ISBN 0-7506-9986-8
    1. Medical jurisprudence--United States.   2. Evidence, Expert--United States.
  I. Nakano, Kenneth K. (Kenneth Kenji), 1942–   .
  II. Title.
    [DNLM: 1. Expert Testimony.   2. Forensic Medicine. W 725 T882e 1998]
  KF8964.Z9T78   1998
  347.73'67--DC21
  DNLM/DLC
  for Library of Congress   97-34806
                                                                  CIP

British Library Cataloguing-in-Publication Data
A catalogue record for this book is available from the British Library.

The publisher offers special discounts on bulk orders of this book.
For information, please contact:
Manager of Special Sales
Butterworth–Heinemann
225 Wildwood Avenue
Woburn, MA 01801-2041
Tel: 781-904-2500
Fax: 781-904-2620

For information on all Butterworth–Heinemann publications available,
contact our World Wide Web home page at: http://www.bh.com

10 9 8 7 6 5 4 3 2

Printed in the United States of America

To my wife, Jean K. Tsushima; my sons, Vincent, Gregory, Matthew, and Stephen; and my parents, Edgar and Alice Tsushima
W.T.T.

To my wife, Juanita W. Nakano; my children, Kenji, Kim, Kam, and Kari; and my mother, Kazuko Nakano
K.K.N.

For their loving support of our work and their inspiration, we dedicate this book to them.

Contents

Preface

In days past, physicians were able to go through an entire professional career without having to testify in a courtroom. Today, however, it is increasingly commonplace for doctors to be summoned as witnesses in some form of legal proceedings, whether in a court of law, in arbitration hearings, or in oral depositions. Given the contemporary litigious atmosphere, society is experiencing an upsurge of civil lawsuits, workers' compensation claims, and medical malpractice suits, amounting to what has been referred to as a *litigation explosion* in the past two decades. Health problems are frequently involved in lawsuits, and expertise is required to explain the medical issues of the dispute. Thus, physicians are needed to testify in a wide range of medicolegal cases arising from traffic accidents, industrial injuries, child custody battles, environmental health conditions, product liability issues, and medical maloccurrences.

Physicians are typically ill-prepared for this daunting task and are highly apprehensive about their involvement in a medicolegal case. Few, if any, medical school curricula include focused coursework in legal medicine. Moreover, continuing education offerings that train physicians in matters of law and courtroom testimony are scant. To fill this void, this book introduces basic concepts and procedures in jurisprudence and, of more practical value, familiarizes physicians with the variety of probing questions encountered when testifying in legal hearings. Some of the most valuable resources in this book are the abundant samples of courtroom testifying, including carefully thought-out responses to cross-examination juxtaposed with examples of hasty and ineffectual answers to the same questions. We present typical challenges in various legal arenas, including personal injury cases, workers' compensation, and medical malpractice claims. Specific forensic issues, such as the scientific bases of expert opinions, and suggestions for effective testifying are emphasized throughout the chapters. The reader of this book will become more aware of the various strategies used by attorneys in court, less intimidated by the ominous environs of the legal world, and better prepared to provide effective medical testimony for the triers of fact.

Originally conceived as a handbook for physicians, residents, and medical students, this text will be useful for other health care professionals, attorneys specializing in the medicolegal area, and law students interested in medical issues.

This book is intended to provide medical education only and is not a rendering of legal or other professional services. The helpfulness of the many suggestions contained here will depend on the specific situation and region relevant to the reader. If legal advice is desired, the reader should obtain the services of a qualified attorney who is familiar with all of the laws of the jurisdiction where the reader practices medicine.

W.T.T.
K.K.N.

Acknowledgments

We are grateful to those who helped us with this book. We acknowledge Dr. Martin Samuels, who gave helpful advice at various phases of our writing. We thank Fran Smith and Jackie Pascua, medical librarians at Straub Clinic, for their assistance with this project, as well as others in the past. Finally, we express our indebtedness to the many attorneys who have grilled us in depositions and at trials over the years. Without our vivid memories of how they artfully and tenaciously cross-examined us, this book could not have been completed.

1

Medicine and Expert Witnessing

The roots of medicine and of law date back to the earliest civilizations of the world, but the formal relationships between these two ancient disciplines are comparatively recent. There are isolated instances of medical doctors being involved with legal procedures, such as when the Roman physician Antistius identified, among the 23 stab wounds of Julius Caesar, the single fatal knife wound to the thorax. However, there is no documentation of physicians being given legal responsibilities in the Western world until the thirteenth century in Bologna, Italy.[1] The earliest medical witness in England appeared in the seventeenth century, with the introduction of scientists as medical police or doctor-detectives.[2] In America, it was not until the nineteenth century that the role of the expert medical witness became visible.[3]

Although the contribution of medicine to the solution of legal problems has been clearly established for over a century, until relatively recently physicians typically were able to conclude their professional careers without ever having to appear in the deliberations of a court. Since about 1970, however, there has been an exponential increase in the number of legal suits filling the court dockets, with spouses suing spouses, workers suing employers, drivers suing drivers, and patients suing doctors in a cultural revolution referred to by some as "the litigation explosion."[4] Statistics for New York state have indicated that payouts in lawsuits against physicians and hospitals have increased 300-fold in 20 years. The National Center for the State Courts reported that a total of 197 million civil cases were filed in the United States in 1992, while an additional 273,000 cases were filed in federal courts.[5]

Because 60–80% of the litigation in U.S. civil courts involves medical evidence,[6] the legal system demands the involvement of medical professionals to explain the technical aspects of the case that are not familiar to the average juror. Some physicians choose to become forensic specialists and voluntarily enter the jurisprudence arena as expert witness, but many physicians whose career choice is to provide health care services are involuntarily subpoenaed to participate in legal procedures as witnesses, to report in court what they have observed and done as a treating physician for a person involved in a lawsuit. In light of the litigious atmosphere prevalent in today's society, many more physicians can expect to be compelled to testify in court because of the pertinent knowledge they possess with regard to the case.[7]

Who Is an Expert Witness?

Physicians may appear in court as an ordinary witness, as an expert witness, or sometimes as both. Any person is an ordinary witness (also known as a *fact witness, material witness, percipient witness,* or *nonexpert witness*) when he or she provides testimony about facts or events he or she has observed. Except for persons who are considered incompetent because of mental impairment or immaturity, generally any adult of sound mind is permitted to appear as a witness. A treating physician is a fact witness on matters related to the patient if the patient's medical condition is at issue in litigation. In such cases, the physician is required to appear as a fact witness and can expect to collect only the normal witness fee for travel, usually amounting to several dollars a day, rather than what is charged for appearing as an expert witness. However, patients or their attorneys often consider a higher fee for the physician witness to elicit the cooperation of the physician to provide testimony.[8]

The definition of an expert witness is, by law, a fairly well-delineated concept, yet is misunderstood by many. In the midst of the "trial of the century," *People v. O.J. Simpson,* the defense called as a witness Robert Huizenga, MD, a Los Angeles specialist in internal medicine. Regarding Mr. Simpson's rheumatoid arthritis condition, Huizenga was asked if he would defer to the opinion of a pre-eminent expert who was a Stanford University professor and author of a standard textbook on rheumatoid arthritis. Huizenga would not yield, and quipped that there are many definitions of an expert and that he had heard as a Harvard University medical student that an expert was "a bastard from Boston with slides." In a court of law, an expert is defined more precisely.

According to Rule 702 of the Federal Rules of Evidence, an expert is a person who, because of specialized "knowledge, skill, experience, training, or education," may provide testimony to "assist the trier of fact to understand the evidence, or to determine a fact in issue."[9] Thus, the expert must be knowledgeable with the scientific literature in the area of expertise and have the ability to explain technical information in a clear and comprehensible manner. Although fact witnesses are permitted to testify only to facts they have observed, the expert witness is allowed to state an opinion on matters in which the average layperson would be unable to understand the facts of the case. In this regard, a physician is the quintessential expert witness in offering professional opinions based on specialized training, education, experience, and skill in the medical sciences. Judges have consistently accepted any person with an MD degree as a medical expert, even one who is not a specialist in the particular condition that is being disputed.[6]

Frequently an outside physician has had no clinical contact with the patient in the usual course of medical care for a condition but may be retained as a medical expert witness to testify on the basis of an independent medical examination, including an examination of the patient and a thorough review of all of the patient's medical records. On some occasions, the nontreating witness, without any examination of the patient, will provide testimony based on a records review or on information presented, such as an undisputed fact or a hypothetical question. On other occasions the outside expert will insist on a thorough examination of the patient before rendering an opinion. Finally, the outside witness is also permitted to testify on the basis of books, treatises, or other information that a specialist would normally use to form an opinion. (It should be noted that some medical experts are retained by attorneys but do not testify. These are experts who are consultants throughout the litigation process, helping lawyers to understand the medical issues of the case and to cross-examine the opposing medical experts.) Whereas the treating physician is legally obligated to testify about the treatment of the plaintiff-patient, the outside expert cannot be compelled to appear in court and testifies voluntarily at the behest of one side in the lawsuit.

As stated earlier, a treating physician who is only a fact witness can merely report what diagnosis and treatment have been provided, as well as other observations made in connection with the patient. However, on many occasions the treating physician, with sufficient professional credentials and a comprehensive knowledge of the case, may also qualify as an expert witness, rendering professional opinions about the cause of the medical condition, the severity of any medical impairment or disability, and the prognosis for the condition. Thus, in the O.J. Simpson example, Dr. Huizenga, who had conducted a physical examination of the defendant, was right in not deferring to the "pre-eminent expert" who had never examined Mr. Simpson.

In recent years, organized medicine has initiated efforts to develop specific guidelines regarding expert witnesses. The American Academy of Pediatrics, the American College of Obstetricians and Gynecologists, the American Academy of Orthopaedic Surgeons, and the American Association of Neurological Surgeons have developed guidelines on the duties of an expert witness.[10–13] In March 1989, the Council of Medical Specialty Societies published its recommended qualifications for physician witnesses and guidelines for expert witness testimony. In addition, the American Medical Association (AMA) Council on Ethical and Judicial Affairs articulated the professional duties of physicians to provide credible medical testimony in court for the protection of the legal rights of both patients and physicians.[14] The AMA has also developed model legislation setting forth minimal criteria for courts to consider in qualifying medical experts. All of these efforts are aimed at ensuring the proper representation of important medical issues in the courtroom.[15]

In Uncharted Territory

As strangers in a strange land, physician witnesses in the courtroom are invariably nervous; some are panic-stricken. Physicians have had practically no medical school exposure to legal medicine or any week-long intensive course in forensic testifying, and they probably experience a form of culture shock when encountering the unfamiliar surroundings and procedures of the courtroom, a place referred to by some forensic medical authorities as "foreign country."[16]

The center stage presence of the court reporter sensitizes the witness to the fact that each word uttered during the trial is being duly recorded. On any occasion, microphones, tape recorders, and video cameras will have an impact on one's self-consciousness and otherwise natural speech and reactions. Add to that the raising of the right hand and swearing an oath to tell the whole truth, and medical witnesses find themselves in circumstances unparalleled in any other situation in their lives. This is no sanctuary of the clinical domain and no familiar emergency room or operating room; this is definitely a courtroom.

Although learned in the technical terms of medicine, the physician witness has to adjust to courtroom language. Physicians will be confused by different usages of ordinary words, such as "treatment" or "treating physician," and will be uncertain about what "certainty" means. In the courtroom, *treatment* refers to any clinical service provided in the care of a patient, including diagnostic work and consultations. Thus, radiologists and pathologists, who usually view themselves as ancillary physicians, will have to answer "Yes" to the question, "Did you have an occasion to treat the plaintiff?" as well as provide dates of treatment for a person with whom they have had no direct contact. Nontreating physicians are those who are retained as expert witnesses to perform independent medical examinations purely for forensic purposes or those who testify after reviewing medical records or learned treatises.

A considerably more significant legal term that needs to be clearly understood is the phrase *reasonable medical certainty*. In the medical realm, there are some occasions in which the physician is unequivocally certain, as with an x-ray film of a fractured bone. At other times, the physician is fairly confident about the diagnosis or prognosis but would not commit to being certain, even if the probability of being correct is high (e.g., 75% or better). In the courtroom, the physician will be asked whether the opinion expressed is to a "reasonable degree of medical certainty." The phrase "reasonable medical certainty" means "more likely than not." In other words, if there is a preponderance—51% or more—of evidence in one direction, then the phrase "reasonable medical certainty" is applicable.[17]

Some physicians mistakenly interpret certainty to mean absolute certainty or the scientific statistical significance of 95–99% probability, whereas reasonable certainty is a much less stringent and exacting standard. Reasonable certainty suggests that the amount of evidence is slightly more weighted on one side than the other. To some, this standard may be too liberal and makes it possible to rationalize any opinion. Nonetheless, medical witnesses must abide by this requirement, and to invoke one's own high level scientific standard would be unfair in a lawsuit.[18] At times, the phrase "reasonable medical probability" is used, which is likely to be better understood by physician witnesses. Because the criteria for reasonable medical certainty may be ambiguous in some jurisdictions, the witness should clarify the definition of this term with an attorney in the appropriate state or jurisdiction.

Finally, the stranger in the courtroom has to adapt to the culture of the jurisprudence system, in particular, the adversarial process in the search for truth. In the medical setting, the physician consults with other health professionals in a collegial exchange of opinions in the pursuit of truth. Clinicians work in alliance with each other to test hypotheses, discover evidence, and reach vital conclusions about a case, guided by their medical school training and the Hippocratic Oath. In sharp contrast, the court system consists of two opposing sides, each gathering support for one side of a legal dispute and attempting to prove that its position alone is true, and that the position of the opposing side is wrong. Thus, whereas professionals in a medical setting may respectfully differ with each other, a cross-examining attorney takes an adversarial position and will not be as cordial. The more experienced and astute lawyer will make every attempt to aggressively expose flaws in the witness's clinical examination, in the quality of the evidence gathered, in the reasoning process involved, and even in the qualifications and character of the physician witness, especially when the medical testimony goes favorably. The physician should expect an adversarial line of questioning, if not an attack, by the opposing lawyer. The intensely critical cross-examination in the courtroom is both unfriendly and foreign to the physician, and for some it is reason enough to avoid the courtroom if at all possible.

Characteristics of a Medical Witness

Because physicians, as a whole, are untrained in courtroom testifying, who then is a good medical witness? Clearly, there is no single ideal medical witness who would be effective before any group of jurors and testifying on any medicolegal issue. The best expert, for example, is not necessarily the best expert witness. In different trial settings different medical knowledge and skill sets, ages, sexes, racial and ethnic backgrounds, and personality styles are likely to be pertinent, but certain qualities have been widely accepted as desirable in an expert witness.[19,20]

A good medical witness should have

1.   The relevant professional qualifications and expertise as documented by an American Board certification and affiliation with specialty organizations. Being a member of an academic faculty of a major institution, actively conducting research, and authoring published papers are considered very impressive.

2.   A fundamental understanding of the legal process and the strategies employed by attorneys in the courtroom.

3.   The ability to communicate complex medical issues in concise and understandable lay terms to the jury.

4.   Calmness and even temperament, with a reasonable and balanced approach to testifying.

5.   Obvious qualities of credibility and forthrightness.

6.   The ability to think quickly on one's feet and thrive on the mental challenges of expert testifying.

7.   The resilience to withstand rigorous cross-examination without being argumentative or adversarial.

8.   The flexibility to adapt to the vicissitudes and time constraints of the judicial system as well as to the language and culture of the courtroom.

9.   The strength to be objective and to avoid being influenced by the protagonistic atmosphere of the courtroom, and to avoid becoming a partisan for one side of the case. The medical opinions are consistent regardless of whether one is testifying for the plaintiff or the defense.

10.   Awareness of the profound importance of medical testimony, which can affect the monetary compensation of injured parties or the reputation of individuals.

The undesirable characteristics of a medical witness are likewise also apparent. Thus, a bad expert witness is one who

1.   Has inadequate qualifications, with credentials that do not measure up to the technical issues of the case, and who is unwilling to acknowledge his or her professional limitations.

2.   Is insensitive to the requirements of the legal system and shows obvious discomfort being around attorneys or appearing at legal hearings.

3.   Insists on spouting obtuse medical jargon and is unable to speak in clear, understandable language to the lay jurors. Furthermore, the witness is prone to verbosity, rambling tangentially with much more

than what is being asked, and losing the jurors' attention and understanding of the relevant medical issues.

4.   Is prone to excitability and dramatics, with an emotional and argumentative approach to testifying.

5.   Appears untrustworthy, unconvincing, and uncertain.

6.   Needs time to react to questions and feels threatened by probing questions.

7.   Has no tolerance for critical questioning and responds with defensiveness, anger, or a condescending attitude toward the court.

8.   Adamantly insists that the court system conform with a physician's medical routines and arrogantly perceives legal proceedings as an intrusive waste of valuable time.

9.   Is consumed by the adversarial nature of litigations and assumes an advocacy role for one side of the case. Displays obvious partisanship with one side of the legal dispute and is impervious to evidence that is inconsistent with his or her point of view.

10.   Is oblivious to the significance of medical testifying, which can seriously damage the lives and reputations of individuals.

What Attorneys Consider

Several other factors enter into the equation when attorneys consider specific expert witness qualities for tactical purposes. These factors include

1.   Availability of the physician witness

2.   Academic physician versus practicing clinician

3.   Professional witness versus average physician

4.   Nationally renowned expert versus local physician

5.   Previously retained expert

6.   Expert who previously testified for opposing side

7.   Age and health of the expert

An attorney's decisions must be governed by practical considerations. Because there are varied time-consuming responsibilities for the expert witness, it is essential that the physician witness be available to evaluate the patient and review the medical documents thoroughly, to participate in trial preparations, to provide oral depositions, and to testify at trial. If your schedule does not permit such involvement or if you will be out of town and unavailable for the various phases of the litigation procedures, you should not accept the responsibilities of an expert witness.

In certain instances, the attorney may prefer as an expert witness a physician who is a full-time professor and researcher. Academicians have the reputation of being highly knowledgeable in their fields and skillful in the verbal presentations of their ideas. Clinicians, on the other hand, have the advantage of being "in the trenches" and able to provide some real-world experiential insights.

Many attorneys choose to employ physicians who regularly engage in forensic cases, so-called professional witnesses, because of their experience and confidence in the courtroom. Their established track record as expert witnesses leaves less to chance and unpredictable testimonies, but it may also present a distasteful image of being a professional hired gun. Thus, in some cases, the attorney will prefer the average physician, whose opinion would appear less slick and rehearsed, less tainted by any biases, and more credible.

Lawyers often believe that jurors are swayed by the appearance of an out-of-town expert with a national reputation. Indeed, physicians with name recognition are held in awe and will have an enormous advantage of being implicitly accepted as a medical authority. At the same time, some jurors may resent the implication that an outsider is needed to edify the local folks. In those circumstances, attorneys will lean toward a hometown doctor whose words, spoken in the same regional idiom and accent as the average jury member, may seem more trustworthy. Following a "locality rule," some jurisdictions require that the expert medical witness in malpractice cases be familiar with the standards of care in the community in which the defendant practices, or at least practices in a locality similar to the defendant.[21]

The use of a previously retained expert has advantages similar to those of using a physician witness who regularly serves as a forensic expert. The attorney will be familiar with the physician's strengths and style as a witness, leaving less opportunity for surprises and unknown factors to arise. On the down side for the previously retained expert will be the impression of being a hired gun for the same law firm. The opposing attorney will ask the number of times an expert has worked for a particular law firm and will try to convey an "arrangement," "allegiance," or "friendship."

Lawyers may want to call on an expert who previously testified for the opposing counsel. Such an individual will be aware of the tactical methods of the opposing attorney and thus better able to cope with the cross-examination. An expert who previously testified for the other side may also be seen as more independent and objective and not favoring one side or the other in a case. Ideally it is best for experts to testify on both plaintiff and defense sides on different occasions.

Attorneys believe that jurors can be affected by the age and health of the expert witness. A middle-aged healthy physician may have the optimal advantage, with the appearance of having substantial medical experience. A youthful physician will be seen as having the most up-to-date medical knowledge but probably lacking in sufficient learning experience. An elderly physician can be perceived as having an abundance of experience and wisdom but, if ailing in any way, may fail to have the positive influence on the jury that a more robust witness would have.

Can Anyone Be an Expert?

How does the court decide who is truly an expert? Can any physician testify about any medical theory or technique, no matter how unusual? Without clear guidelines, there would be concerns that jurors will be hearing opinions that lack scientific validity, drawing incorrect conclusions, and determining unjust outcomes in legal cases. Since 1923, the Federal Appellate decision in *Frye v. United States*[22] has provided the needed ground rules to ensure that an expert witness's opinion is based on *generally accepted* scientific principles rather than on idiosyncratic theories or "junk science." In the Frye case, the U.S. Court of Appeals for the District of Columbia rejected a systolic blood pressure deception test, a predecessor of the modern polygraph lie detector, and decided that a scientific technique must be "sufficiently established to have gained general acceptance in the particular field in which it belongs" before an expert opinion based on that technique is admissible into evidence.

Adopted by Congress in 1975, the codified Federal Rules of Evidence (cf. Appendix A), specifically Rule 702, provide that qualified experts are allowed to testify about scientific, technical, or other specialized knowledge if their testimony "will assist" the triers of fact in understanding the evidence or to determine a fact in issue. Since the Federal Rules have been introduced, lawyers have debated whether the more liberal rules' "helpful and reliable" standard has supplanted the Frye rule's "general acceptance" standard, although published decisions indicate that in practice there have been no marked differences between these two approaches.[23]

In 1993, based on the case of *Daubert v. Merrell Dow Pharmaceuticals*, the U.S. Supreme Court established the most current standard regarding the admissibility of scientific evidence.[24] The Daubert case attracted considerable interest regarding junk science[25] being presented in federal courts, as evidenced by the filing of 22 amicus curiae briefs, including one by the AMA. The trial court in the Daubert case refused to consider expert testimony for the plaintiffs that Bendectin could cause serious birth defects when ingested by a woman during pregnancy because the work of these experts had not been subjected to peer review and had not been shown to be "generally accepted or reliable" by the scientific community. The Supreme Court held that the adoption of the Federal Rules of Evidence superseded the Frye test, replacing it with a more liberal rule that permits the admission of a much greater range of expert evidence without permitting the admission of everything claiming to be scientific knowledge.

With the Daubert decision, the Supreme Court emphasized that it is the responsibility of federal judges to review expert evidence to ensure that it rests on a reliable foundation and is relevant to the case. The Court suggested that, in performing this function, judges should consider the following factors to determine the admissibility of expert testimony:

1.   Whether it has been tested using some accepted scientific methodology;

2.   Whether it has been subject to peer review and journal publication;

3.   Whether the known or potential rate of error of the scientific technique justifies its use; and

4.   Whether it has achieved a degree of acceptance within the scientific community.

The Daubert decision, in effect, eliminates the 70-year-old Frye rule and permits a broader admission of expert opinion, even when it has not achieved a large measure of acceptability within the profession itself. Physicians who appear as expert witnesses in court should be well acquainted with the 1993 Supreme Court decision, which has resulted in what has become known as the Daubert test or Daubert standard of evidence admissibility. Because the judge has wide discretion over who will be accepted as an expert, ultimately an expert witness is one whom the judge deems to be an expert witness.

Closing Arguments

The rising number of civil lawsuits today and the increased need for medical expertise in the courtroom heighten the chances that a physician will be summoned to testify in a legal hearing. In some cases, the physician is merely a fact witness reporting what has been observed and recorded in the course of treating a person involved in litigation. More often than not, the treating physician by virtue of technical training and credentials is also considered an expert witness who is permitted to offer professional opinions about the cause, related symptoms, and prognosis of the patient's medical condition. Others considered as expert witnesses include nontreating physicians who conduct independent medical examinations specifically for forensic purposes or medical specialists who testify based on a review of the patient's records or standard textbooks. In short, physicians are experts in the courtroom when they can provide medical, scientific, and related knowledge and understanding beyond the ken of the average lay juror.

For most physicians, the act of testifying in court is a trial in itself. Strangers in a strange land, physicians are intimidated by the unfamiliar environs of the courtroom, with its rigid formalities, idiosyncratic rules, and technical language. Superimposed over all of this is the adversarial system in the discovery of truth, with medical witnesses having to run a gauntlet of incisive questioning. The physician's credentials can be attacked and the medical testimony subjected to harsh inquisition and possible ridicule. To survive this ominous process, physicians now and in the future will have to become familiar with the legal system as our society moves even further into litigious waters.

There is no ideal medical witness, but the bare minimum requirements are that the expert has the relevant professional qualifications and the ability to clearly communicate the technical issues of the case. The courtroom is not for everyone, certainly not for the faint of heart. But with sufficient preparation and useful road maps, almost every physician can be a good witness, and the challenging journey of testifying in court can be professionally stimulating and personally rewarding.

References

1. Gee DJ, Mason JK. *The Courts and the Doctor*. Oxford, England: Oxford University Press, 1990.
2. Jones CAG. *Expert Witnesses: Science, Medicine and the Practice of Law*. Oxford, England: Clarendon Press, 1994.
3. Mohr JC. *Doctors and the Law: Medical Jurisprudence in Nineteenth Century America*. New York: Oxford University Press, 1993.
4. Olson WK. *The Litigation Explosion: Understanding the Legal Revolution*. New York: Truman Talley Books/Plume, 1993.
5. Menendez K. *Taming the Lawyers*. Santa Monica, CA: Merritt Publishing, 1996.
6. Horsley JE. *Testifying in Court: A Guide for Physicians* (4th ed). Los Angeles: Product Management Information Corp, 1992.
7. Shuman DW. Testimonial compulsion: the involuntary medical witness. *J Legal Med* 1983;4:419–446.
8. Dunn JD. Medical Testimony: Physician as Witness. In American College of Legal Medicine (ed), *Legal Medicine: Legal Dynamics of Medical Encounters* (2nd ed). St. Louis: Mosby–Year Book, 1991;535–540.
9. Moore JW. *Moore's Federal Practice: Federal Rules of Evidence*. New York: Matthew Bender, 1985.
10. American College of Pediatrics Committee on Medical Liability. Guidelines for expert witness testimony. *Pediatrics* 1989;83:312–313.
11. American College of Obstetricians and Gynecologists. *Ethical Issues Related to Expert Testimony by Obstetricians and Gynecologists*. Washington, DC: American College of Obstetricians and Gynecologists, 1987.
12. American Academy of Orthopaedic Surgeons. *Qualification and Guidelines for the Orthopaedic Expert Witness*. Park Ridge, IL: American Academy of Orthopaedic Surgeons, 1989.
13. American Association of Neurological Surgeons, Ethics and Human Values Committee. *Testimony in Professional Liability Cases*. Park Ridge, IL: American Association of Neurological Surgeons, 1987.
14. American Medical Association. *Current Opinions of the Council on Ethical and Judicial Affairs*. Chicago: AMA, 1987.
15. American Medical Association, Department of State Legislation. *Model legislation to provide for the regulation of expert witnesses in medical malpractice injury actions*. October 1989.
16. Appelbaum PS, Gutheil TG. *Clinical Handbook of Psychiatry and the Law* (2nd ed). Baltimore: Williams & Wilkins, 1991.
17. American College of Legal Medicine. *Legal Medicine: Legal Dynamics of Medical Encounters* (2nd ed). St. Louis: Mosby–Year Book, 1991.
18. Liebenson HA. *You, the Expert Witness*. Mundelein, IL: Callaghan & Company, 1962.

19. Vevaina JR, Finz LL. The Expert Witness in Medical Malpractice Litigation. In JR Vevaina, RC Bone, E Kassoff (eds), *Legal Aspects of Medicine*. New York: Springer-Verlag, 1989;33–38.
20. Reynolds MP, King PSD. *The Expert Witness and His Evidence* (2nd ed). London: Blackwell Scientific, 1992.
21. Quimby CW Jr. General Considerations of Medical Testimony. In AE James (ed), *Legal Medicine: With Special Reference to Diagnostic Imaging*. Baltimore: Urban & Schwarzenberg, 1980;49–61.
22. *Frye v. U.S.*, 293 F 1013, 334 ALR 145 (D.C. Cir 1923).
23. Ayala FJ, Black B. Science and the courts. *Am Sci* 1993;81:230–239.
24. *Daubert v. Merrell Dow Pharmaceuticals*, 113 SCt 2786, 61 LW 4805, 1993.
25. Huber PW. *Galileo's Revenge: Junk Science in the Courtroom*. New York: Basic Books, 1991.

2

Preparation for Trial and Presentation in Court

Theodoric Beck in his presidential address delivered before his medical colleagues in New York surprised his audience by choosing among the various professional issues of the day the topic of medical evidence in the court of justice. Because insufficient attention had been paid to the role of medical experts in the courtrooms, Beck offered the following pieces of advice:

1. With respect to the use of professional language, some medical and scientific terms are essential for accuracy, but try to state the facts plainly and directly. Do not try to dazzle the jury with pedantic showmanship.

2. Stand firm by your testimony. Do not yield to an aggressive cross-examining attorney.

3. Take careful notes when performing a forensic examination as an expert and refer to the notes in court. Notes help to maintain consistency in the testimony and prevent the witness from misstating the findings.

4. When appropriate, bring a standard textbook to refer to while on the witness stand.

5.   Take seriously the concept of the whole truth. Avoid being partisan and share all the facts you have, even those that may not be favorable to the side who summoned you.

6.   Medical witnesses should treat each other with respect. Public battles between physicians do not serve the judicial process and embarrass the medical profession.

Beck's address to his fellow physicians was delivered on February 2, 1828, but his words of wisdom are timeless and are as apropos today as they were in his time.[1] And as in 1828, there continues to be a dearth of material to guide the medical doctor through the uncharted course of the jurisprudence system. Few if any medical schools include legal medicine as a routine course in their curricula, and textbooks on the interface of medicine and law are rarely published. A small number of books that offer guidance to potential medical witnesses is listed in an annotated bibliography found in Appendix B and was a rich source of the practical advice that is presented throughout this book.

General Guides for the Medical Witness

The difficulties of being a medical witness are a function of the unknown territory of the legal system. It may be courageous to accept the challenge of a perilous journey; it is foolhardy to proceed without a map. The following three chapters are, in essence, some useful landmarks for guiding the physician toward the goal of providing effective courtroom testimony, including (1) preparation for trial, (2) presentation in court, (3) direct examination, and (4) cross-examination. The first two topics are the focus of this chapter. Chapters 3 and 4 cover the direct examination and the cross-examination, respectively.

Preparation for Trial

The legal system seemingly moves at glacial speed, and it is often presumed that there is a surplus of time to prepare for a trial. However, given the hectic professional schedules of most physicians, it is easy to set aside a court-related case for several weeks, months, and sometimes a year or more, only to be suddenly informed that the important trial date has arrived. Because many health professionals fail to take sufficient measures to prepare for testifying, expert witnesses notoriously present vague, garbled, and inadequate testimony.[2] Proper pretrial preparation consists of a review of medical records, reports, and relevant scientific literature, appropriate communications with the attorney, and preparing court exhibits. Medical witnesses should request a complete set of relevant documents from the attorney and make sure that all materials have been provided.

As the designated expert regarding a particular case, you should expect to testify regarding the nature and extent of the patient's injuries or disease, the treatment provided, the pain and suffering experienced, and the prognosis. You must do your homework and be thoroughly familiar with the many details of the case, not merely the results of the clinical examination, but the patient's previous medical history and the findings of other physicians, especially those who have been employed by the opposing side as expert medical specialists to present a contrary point of view. Even though you may have a tenable position with a solid foundation of evidence, if you report inaccurately in court details, such as laboratory results, or if you are unaware of inconsistent data, your credibility as a witness will be diminished.

You must be sensitive not only to the strengths of your findings but also to the weak areas in the case, such as any conflicting results or explanations. It would be of value for you to place yourself in the position of the adversary expert to identify all of the weaknesses and the controversial issues in the case.[3] Do not write down anything (e.g., speculations) that you would not want everyone to see. Your notes are discoverable and must be made available to the adverse side. If you have not seen the patient for several weeks, you may desire a checkup visit to update your knowledge of the patient's status, particularly if the medical condition has changed.[4] Finally, you need to have a sufficient grasp of the scientific literature pertinent to the case.

After you feel well prepared with the issues of the case, then you must share your knowledge with the attorney. You may have to adjust the level of your communication of the technical information depending on the attorney, whose medical sophistication may range from being totally naive to being a highly experienced lawyer who has litigated numerous medicolegal cases. These days you may even encounter the occasional attorney who is also a medical or nursing school graduate.

Each lawyer will, on the basis of what the client has said or what he or she gleans from the medical records, develop a reasonable medical explanation about the case, which may or may not be valid. Your job is to explain the scientific realities of the case so that the attorney becomes fully educated about the facts and the ramifications of the medical evidence. The attorney, in turn, will establish the limits of the area you as the expert will address. With your assistance, the attorney can prepare the most effective way to present your findings and conclusions.

Discuss the fee arrangements with the attorney. Indicate that you will be charging for reviewing documents, writing a report, doing research requested by the attorney, and testifying at a deposition and in court. Physicians usually charge hourly fees rather than an estimated total amount, and the hourly fee is often higher than the usual office visit because of the preparation time, the logistics in arranging legal activities, and the generally arduous nature of expert testifying. Clarify, preferably in writing, whether the attorney or the patient will be billed. It is, of course, unethical for physicians to arrange for compensation that is contingent on the outcome of the litigation.[5]

Because of the busy schedules kept by both doctors and lawyers, it will be easy to minimize communications and reduce them to brief telephone calls. This is not advisable. There is no substitute for a face-to-face meeting with a mutual sharing of documents, reports, and opinions. The attorney needs to know from you what the quality of the medical evidence is as well as how you think and react. Likewise, it will be helpful for you to know how the attorney perceives the case and what is expected from your expert testimony. The experienced litigator will familiarize the witness with basic matters, such as the mechanics of the legal process, as well as the pivotal legal issues, the strengths and weaknesses of the case, and anticipated lines of cross-examination.[6] The attorney can assist the expert in responding to difficult questions or reconciling apparent inconsistencies in the medical records. Some believe that it is advantageous to present any weaknesses (e.g., the absence of important tests) during the direct examination, rather than trying to cope with these unfavorable issues in cross-examination. In this way, you can demonstrate your awareness of the problem and your consideration of it in drawing your conclusions.[7] Any potential damage presented by this issue would thus be minimized.

With respect to communicating with attorneys, it must be stressed that discussions with the referring lawyer must be very limited *before* your formulation of an opinion, so that you can affirm that your opinion was reached without undue influence from the attorney.[7] Thorough consultations with the referring attorney should be conducted *after* your opinion has been determined, the date of the examination, the written report, and the attorney consultation. In preparing your testimony, it is wise to discuss in advance the kinds of questions and even the sequence of questions that will best present your opinions. While you can collaborate with the lawyer about the questions to be asked, all answers must be yours and yours alone.

Everyone agrees that a witness should be impartial and objective. This is more easily said than done. When working closely with an attorney, an emotional alliance can develop that could cause you to ignore or reject possible interpretations that are inconsistent with the attorney's views. You could feel that acknowledging the alternative viewpoint is a form of disloyalty and betrayal. Medical experts should be aware of this possibility and must conscientiously adhere to the duty to be nonpartisan and objective; failure to do so can result in a miscarriage of justice.

Organize your thoughts and be prepared with detailed answers for the obligatory questions about diagnosis, prognosis, and the like. Do not, however, memorize your testimony, because you can be easily distracted, lose your train of thought, and appear confused. An overly prepared speech may seem rehearsed and insincere.

The task of expert testifying is not unlike giving a medical lecture. The purpose is to teach, and you achieve this end not only with an organized verbal presentation but by strategic use of various visual exhibits. Witnesses can bring to court photographs, slides, drawings, charts, graphs, plastic models, medical equipment, and other visual aids to augment the oral testimony. Jurors find it difficult to visualize medical information, and their understanding is greatly enhanced by a vivid illustration of your findings. You must realize that it requires time and forethought to organize high-quality exhibits for trial purposes. For the juror, these visual aids are not only worth a thousand words, but they also provide mental images that are often better retained than a lengthy verbal testimony.

As a medical witness, whether you are the treating physician or an expert retained specifically to testify in the case, a court writ, known as a *subpoena duces tecum,* will be served on you, commanding you to appear with records and testify before a particular judge on a prescribed day at an exact time. You must cooperate with the subpoena, regardless of other professional obligations. If you are unable to appear to testify at the designated time, such as being out of town, the court may be able to reschedule you at a more convenient time, or your sworn testimony could be taken by a court reporter via a videotaped deposition with the attorneys from both sides present. In any event, it should be kept in mind that the court has the authority to compel your attendance no matter how inconvenient it may be to you. At times, if you have agreed with the attorney to serve as a witness, no subpoena will be issued, and arrangements can be made for you to appear in court with minimal interruption in your schedule.

In certain circumstances, a subpoena may be necessary. Sometimes a physician, for a variety of reasons, is highly reluctant to appear in court. This is especially true if the physician is being called by the side opposed to his or her patient or if testimony is requested against a medical colleague or hospital. The physician who fails to respond to a subpoena is in contempt of court and may face severe punishment including, although rarely, incarceration.

A few words about *confidentiality* are in order. As you prepare for testifying, you may anticipate being asked questions about matters that have been regarded as confidential communication between yourself and your patient. Most states today have statutes that specifically protect the privileged communications between doctor and patient, that is, no disclosure of privileged matter is permitted without the patient's consent.[8]

If your patient waives the privilege to confidentiality, you will be obligated to disclose the information requested. When you are asked to testify on behalf of the patient, the request functions as a waiver of the privilege. However, if you are called as a witness for the side opposing your patient, the patient can claim the privilege by objections to your testifying or answering questions about any confidential matter. If the patient's lawyer does not object to your testimony, the privilege is considered waived.[8]

Although specific legal mandates vary among the states, there are identifiable exceptions to privileged communications, especially those involving psychiatric issues. For example, at a psychiatric commitment hearing, the psychiatrist must testify when there is a threat of imminently dangerous activity by the patient against self or others. In a criminal sanity hearing, the psychiatrist who performs the court-ordered examination will be testifying about what is said and should provide a detailed, comprehensive warning, preferably in writing, that communications during the examination are not privileged. Another common exception to privileged communication occurs in civil cases when a person has invoked a mental or emotional condition as an element of one's claim in a lawsuit. In these cases the judge usually finds that justice demands the disclosure of psychotherapy sessions because it would be unfair to the other side to prevent such information from being heard.

Finally, as the trial date nears, you must clear your work schedule, allowing ample time to travel to the courthouse, find parking, and locate the courtroom. If this is your first experience with a particular courthouse, you may find it helpful before the court date to go to the court building and familiarize yourself with the locale and the courtroom itself. Arriving late, appearing frazzled by parking problems, or getting lost in the courthouse are not optimal ways to offer oneself as a competent professional. To minimize the waiting time in the courthouse before testifying, it is possible in certain situations to arrange with the lawyer to telephone you when the time for testifying is near.

Some physicians may be leery of the ethics of consulting with the attorney. Discussions with lawyers are not only ethical, they are necessary.[4] The American Medical Association guidelines for forensic testimony recommend that expert witnesses prepare their testimony with the attorney. Justice is best served when the expert has considered all of the relevant medical facts and issues in a case and is thoroughly prepared to present useful testimony for the court. Members of the medical and legal professions recognize that physicians and lawyers are drawn into increasing association as the knowledge and services of both professions are required so that the rights of individuals may be appropriately determined in legal hearings.

Presentation in Court

Going to testify in court is like going to a job interview: you want to put your best foot forward. That is, you want to dress appropriately, be prompt, and conduct yourself in a thoroughly professional manner. Imagine going to a job interview casually dressed, arriving a few minutes late, and creating a less than positive impression with the interviewer. You may, in fact, be the most qualified person for the job, but the manner in which you present yourself will determine whether or not you will be hired.

Arrive at the courthouse before the scheduled time of your appearance. Physicians understandably resent the long waiting period wasted outside the courtroom before taking the witness stand. Many courts are sensitive to the important schedule and clinical responsibilities of physicians and try whenever possible to accommodate them by taking the medical witness out of turn or squeezing the physician's testimony in the middle of someone else's appearance on the witness stand. Although some down time at a trial is unavoidable, the waiting period can be used to make valuable last minute reviews of your notes.

It is never acceptable for physicians to be late for their date in the courtroom. For those witnesses who are served a formal subpoena to report at the courthouse at a specific time, a late arrival may be cause for the judge to fine (or even jail) the witness for contempt of court. Even if no sanction takes place, a tardy arrival will be considered rude and unprofessional by the judge and jurors.

Because of court rules excluding scheduled witnesses from sitting in the courtroom audience, you will probably not be allowed to listen to witnesses who precede you on the witness stand. At times exceptions are made on this "rule on witnesses" to allow expert witnesses to observe what the other experts state in court, but the argument will be made that hearing prior testimony can provide the observer with an unfair advantage in that you could then include in your testimony a rebuttal to previous opposing opinions.[7] You are also warned not to discuss the case with anyone in the hallway, bathroom, or elevator; you never know to whom you are talking or if anyone overhears your comments.

If you reach the courtroom at the designated time but are not called right away, you can ask the attorney through the court bailiff or at the next recess to put you on the witness stand as soon as possible. The attorney will then request the judge to take you out of turn—that is, withdraw the witness whose testimony is still in progress—so that you can testify and return to your office. The judge will usually be amenable to your request.

Your appearance and bearing will affect the jurors' perceptions of your competence as an expert. You should be well groomed (fresh shave, appropriate haircut or hair style, clean hands and fingernails) and you should not chew gum at any time. Your attire should be simple, comfortable, conservative, and professional, such as a dark business suit. Discuss your appearance with the attorney and the biases of the region in which you are testifying. You may bring pertinent records, but do not bring unnecessary items, such as a lunch container or a shopping bag. Unless absolutely necessary, leave your pager or cellular phone at the office, or leave it with the bailiff, who can take messages. Any notes or documents you bring to the witness stand can be marked as an exhibit and admitted into evidence. If there is anything you do not want in the hands of the opposing counsel, such as some hypotheses or speculations you have made, then make certain that they are not brought into the courtroom.

Do not rush into the courtroom. Calmly approach the witness stand with a serious businesslike expression. Viewing the judge and jurors with a wide smile or a worried expression is not appropriate at this point.

The taking of the oath begins your testifying. Say "I do" in a clear and strong voice. Some witnesses are uncertain about the exact meaning of "the truth, the whole truth, and nothing but the truth." Taken literally, it is impossible and impractical to tell "the whole truth" regarding a medical condition, which requires at least a few hours of didactic lecturing. Tell the jury what they need to know, not all that you know.[2] The expert witness may do best with a negative interpretation of the oath, that is, to not intentionally tell an untruth and to not deliberately hide a truth.[9]

Sit upright with a dignified posture in the witness stand, that is, do not slouch or display nervous mannerisms. Look confident and capable. Avoid headshaking, sneering, or eyerolling. You are being constantly observed by jurors,[10] and sometimes videotaped in certain courts. When being asked questions, give undivided attention and maintain eye contact with the attorney. When your answer is lengthy, looking occasionally at the jurors is helpful because they are the primary audience for your testimony.

Listen to each question carefully and completely, and direct your answer to what is being asked, nothing more. Your attorney knows what you need to say on the stand and will ask you follow-up questions that will enable you to express your entire opinion. If you volunteer more information than is needed, you may be yielding more opportunity for attack on your opinions.

If you have to speak to the judge, remember to address the judge as "Your Honor." In a prolonged exchange when the repetition of "Your Honor" becomes awkward, you may also use "Sir" or "Ma'am" to show your respect toward authority. As for the attorneys in court, you should say "Sir" or "Ma'am" or address them as "Mister" or "Ms" to maintain a courteous relationship with them.

Communication is the essence of testifying. Speak clearly into the microphone in everyday language, using technical terms when unavoidable and clarifying medical lingo immediately so that the lay jurors can understand. Words such as "oriented," "trauma," and "hypertension" may be basic vocabulary for health professionals, but the average juror may be uncertain of their specific meanings. An erudite discourse comprised of polysyllabic medical jargon will be beyond the comprehension of the jury and is much less effective than the use of plain English. At the same time do not talk down to them or purposely use poor grammar, which can be offensive to jurors. (Simple language may not be as important when testifying before a judge rather than a jury.)

Speak with confidence and assurance, preferably with an economy of words. Do not answer questions too quickly; it may appear to be a rehearsed act. Rapid or mumbled speech or a soft voice will not be heard by all of the jurors, who may miss an important fact or viewpoint. Speak slowly enough to be understood, but not so deliberately as to be boring. Be aware that hesitation and uncertainty in your voice may raise doubts in the jurors' minds.

You may use written notes when you are testifying, but it is best when you can answer extemporaneously in a natural teaching style. You should be familiar with the information you want to present and should rely on notes as little as possible (e.g., to provide specific facts such as dates and test results).

Your demeanor should be professional, pleasant, and relatively relaxed. Some nervousness is not only expected and acceptable, but it may help you to be more alert and animated while you testify. Furthermore, there are drawbacks to appearing too slick and polished in your presentation.

Avoid appearing pedantic or condescending. Jurors are more receptive to those who show proper respect to them as triers of fact. Avoid also being dogmatic or authoritarian. Be willing to admit that there could be alternative views and conclusions about the case. You are expected to be an impartial expert, not an advocate for your patient, your attorney, or any cause. If anything, be an advocate for the medical truth.

One of the most important traits to present as a witness is your forthrightness and credibility. When you hedge or hesitate or when you avoid giving a direct answer to a question, you appear unsure of yourself and seem untrustworthy. Although you are, in fact, called on by one side of the legal case, you must consciously exercise independent thinking as an objective and responsible expert, with a commitment to honesty.[11] Under vigorous questioning, when you have to defend your qualifications as well as your opinions, it is difficult to remain neutral. As a party to the adversary system, a witness under vigorous cross-examination is tempted to become an advocate for one side. For the sake of justice and your own integrity, you should identify only with your honest opinions and advocate for those opinions. When you appear to be advocating for one side, you will be perceived by jurors as a hired gun and your testimony will be discredited.

Only offer opinions that have solid scientific foundation. Support your conclusions with a clear explanation of the evidence and how your inferences were drawn. Resist a lawyer pressuring you to testify on matters, such as causation or prognosis, that may go beyond the limits of your medical evidence. The jury will appreciate your display of independence rather than being a pawn of the attorney. If you venture beyond the dictates of your data, an experienced cross-examiner will surely pick apart any unfounded opinions and undermine your credibility and value to the case. Regarding any weaknesses in your findings, it may be wise to introduce the vulnerable aspects of your testimony in direct examination, rather than have the opposing counsel expose those flaws in cross-examination. This is an approach you want to discuss with your attorney.

Refer to your records when necessary, as it is difficult to recall the specific dates and many details in a medical case. You should keep in mind the major facts of the case, but it is also acceptable to refresh your memory by checking with your records. This is far better than saying, "I don't remember exactly."[12]

Do not guess if you are not certain. When you do not know the answer, the best response is "I don't know."[13] Recognize the limits of your expertise; you are not expected to know everything in a field as broad and complex as medicine.

Do not answer questions you do not understand. Once you answer a question, it becomes your sworn testimony. Thus, it will be difficult to change your answer later without appearing inconsistent, and a defensive response such as "I misunderstood your question" leaves an unfavorable impression with the jury. If a question is unclear or ambiguous, you can ask the attorney to rephrase the question, but do not make this request too many times. Occasionally it is acceptable to rephrase an awkwardly phrased question: "If you're asking me _____, then my answer is _____."[14]

When the cross-examining lawyer is hostile and sarcastic, it is difficult to remain the calm pacifist. Do not be tempted to debate with the opposing counsel. In the legal arena, you are unlikely to win a battle of wits, and even if you do, you may appear arrogant and adversarial rather than professional and objective.

Is there a role for humor while testifying? Humor in the courtroom can be a double-edged sword. For example,

Q. Doctor, is your appearance here this morning pursuant to a subpoena I sent to your office?

A. No. This is how I usually dress when I go to work.

Timely witticism and laughter can be a refreshing break from an otherwise grim or boring hearing, and a jury who laughs could be establishing rapport with the witness. However, a joke runs the risk of being ill-timed or in poor taste, and perceived as disrespectful, given the serious business of court trials. Thus, humor is a delicate matter that must be used good naturedly with sensitivity and respect for the dignity of the courtroom.[14]

Closing Arguments

The initial guidelines for expert witnesses appear commonsensical: prepare for your testifying, discuss your testimony with the attorney, and present a professional demeanor. It is true that, as the expert in a trial, you know more about medicine than anyone else in the courtroom, but it is dangerous to rest on your laurels and attempt to testify without due diligence to the pretrial preparation needed to perform dutifully on the witness stand. Many physicians unfortunately fail to follow these simple tips, and they provide an unclear explanation of the medical issues, subject themselves to damaging questions about their conclusions, and appear less than competent and credible.

Do your homework; do not try to "wing it." This is much like preparing for any skilled activity, such as in sports or the arts. One must prepare, practice, and perform. Opposing counselors have all the facts and figures at their fingertips and are primed to assail any errors or gaps of information that an unprepared witness exhibits. You may indeed have a better understanding of the technical issues being argued, but if you fail to know precise dates and details, you will appear no more an expert than the average jury member.

Talk with the attorney who is calling on you. Tell your lawyer what you know about the patient and listen to the lawyer's assessment of the critical medicolegal issues involved in the case. Your attorney can be a valued ally in the courtroom, especially when the opposing attorney launches an assault on your testimony, and attorneys can best help you when they are familiar with you and the strengths and weaknesses of your testimony.

To succeed as an expert witness, the physician's medical acumen is simply not enough. The importance of how you present yourself before the jury cannot be overemphasized. Your outward appearance, your professional demeanor, your communications skills, and your honest objectivity are key factors in ensuring your effectiveness on the witness stand. (A brief checklist for expert witnesses is presented in Appendix C.)

References

1. Mohr JC. *Doctors and the Law: Medical Jurisprudence in Nineteenth Century America*. New York: Oxford University Press, 1993.
2. Rossi FF. *Expert Witnesses*. Chicago: American Bar Association, 1991.
3. Matson JV. *Effective Expert Witnessing: A Handbook for Technical Professionals*. Chelsea, MI: Lewis Publishers, 1990.
4. Horsley JE. *Testifying in Court: A Guide for Physicians* (4th ed). Los Angeles: Product Management Information Corp., 1992.
5. Foreman J. Contingency fee for medical expert witness. *Arch Ophthalmol* 1990;108:923.
6. Appelbaum PS, Gutheil TG. *Clinical Handbook of Psychiatry and the Law* (3rd ed). Baltimore: Williams & Wilkins, 1991.
7. Shapiro DL. *Psychological Evaluation and Expert Testimony: A Practical Guide to Forensic Work*. New York: Van Nostrand Reinhold, 1984.
8. Warden KP. Direct Examination. In AE James (ed), *Legal Medicine: With Special Reference to Diagnostic Imaging*. Baltimore: Urban & Schwarzenberg, 1980;75–86.
9. Gee DJ, Mason JK. *The Courts and the Doctor*. Oxford, England: Oxford University Press, 1993.
10. Zobel HB, Rous SN. *Doctors and the Law*. New York: WW Norton, 1993.
11. Katz J. "The Fallacy of the Impartial Expert" revisited. *Bull Am Acad Psychiatry Law* 1992;20:141–152.
12. Liebenson HA. *You, the Expert Witness*. Mundelein, IL: Callaghan & Company, 1962.
13. Moritz AR, Morris RC. *Handbook of Legal Medicine* (4th ed). St. Louis: CV Mosby, 1975.
14. Brodsky SL. *Testifying in Court: Guidelines and Maxims for the Expert Witness*. Washington, DC: American Psychological Association, 1991.

3

Qualifying of the Witness and Direct Examination

The qualifying of the witness and the direct examination constitute the first phase of the expert witness's testifying and commence after the sworn oath is taken. The direct examination is conducted by the attorney who has requested the witness to testify and is a vital part of the testimony in which the medical expert shares technical knowledge about the issues of the case. With appropriate pretrial preparation, you will be able to anticipate the series of questions asked by the attorney to present the desired information in a logically flowing and persuasive manner.

Qualifying the Witness

Testifying begins with the qualifying of the witness, which is a detailed presentation of the physician's training and experience, including:

- Professional education (schools, degrees, dates)
- Internship and residency training (fellowship, apprenticeship)
- Current employment and duties
- Current professional activities (specializations)
- License and board certifications

- Professional memberships
- Research, teaching, and publications
- Honors, recognitions

The qualifying of a physician witness consists of standard questions to verify the doctor's competence to testify, including:

Q. Doctor, could you tell us about your educational background, beginning with your undergraduate studies?

Q. What medical school did you attend?

Q. Where did you receive your residency training in your specialty?

Q. How long did your residency take?

Q. Are you board certified in the field of _____ ?

Q. Tell us what the requirements are for board certification in _____ .

Q. What professional work have you done since you completed your residency?

Q. In what states are you licensed to practice medicine?

Q. What is your current position as a physician?

Q. What professional organizations do you belong to?

The astute attorney wants to bring out some of the unique strengths the physician brings to the courtroom. Questions to highlight the witness's special assets might include:

Q. Have you presented any lectures or workshops in your area of expertise?

Q. Do you do any teaching or supervision?

Q. Have you done any research in your area of specialty?

Q. Do you have any publications in your field?

Q. Have you held an office in any of your medical societies?

Q. What honors or recognitions have you received as a doctor?

After this initial query of a general nature, the attorney may ask about any experience pertaining to the specific medical condition being disputed, as well as prior experience as an expert witness. Examples of such questions are:

Q. In the course of your medical practice, have you treated patients who have _____ disorder?

Q. About how many such patients have you treated?

Q. Have you assisted in court proceedings before by providing expert medical testimony for the court?

Q. On approximately how many occasions have you been accepted as an expert witness in court?

Q. Have you ever been rejected as an expert witness?

The aim here is not simply to show the depth of your training and experience, but how your expertise bears directly on the medical issues of the case.[1] You and your attorney want the jury to be confident with the depth and relevance of your qualifications as an expert medical witness so that they are inclined to accept your opinions. The attorney will try to encompass as many impressive and relevant aspects of your professional background as possible without boring the jury and losing their attention.

You neither want to downplay your authority as a medical expert nor to appear as a pompous show-off.[2] To save time and avoid a tedious litany of all your achievements, memberships, and the like, the attorney may offer your credentials into evidence by submitting your curriculum vitae (CV) as an exhibit that can be available to the jurors for their review during deliberations.

In your CV be careful not to exaggerate any aspect of your professional background. Portray accurately your hospital staff privileges and your involvement as a medical school clinical faculty member. For business and public relations purposes, you may have a resume that generously describes your skills and experiences. You would be wiser to submit for court purposes a CV that is more conservative and not an obvious self-promotion tool. Any attempt to magnify your credentials will be identified and exposed by the opposing attorney and serve as a point of embarrassment for you.

While general guidelines such as the Federal Rules of Evidence and the Daubert standard (discussed in Chapter 1) exist, the courts provide no specific criteria to determine whether a physician is qualified to provide expert medical testimony. In general, a physician's qualification is acknowledged without difficulty if the expert is appropriately licensed and has credentials as a specialist that are commonly accepted as sufficient by medical colleagues.

On occasion, the opposing attorney will object that the physician is not qualified and cannot offer an opinion. The opposing attorney will ask the court to *voir dire* or examine the competency of the witness in an effort to persuade the judge that the physician does not qualify as an expert. The strategy here is to prevent the witness from testifying, and even if the judge qualifies the physician, the voir dire could at least diminish the credibility of the expert witness by emphasizing the physician's lack of credentials or experience.

The opposing lawyer can challenge the physician's qualifications in various ways. If you have taken a marketing approach with your CV, the opposing lawyer might ask questions such as these in a voir dire cross-examination:

Q. You refer to yourself as a physician and surgeon. Do you operate on your patients?

A. Very rarely. But, on the basis of my medical degree, I reserve the right to call myself a physician and surgeon.

Q. Your CV states that you attended Stanford University. What was the extent of your matriculation at Stanford?

A. I had an intensive 6-week training in using laser equipment at Stanford.

Q. Do you actually admit patients at four different hospitals?

A. Well, no. I'm on the active medical staff at two hospitals and on the courtesy staff of the other two.

Q. You say you are on the medical school's clinical faculty. When was the last time you supervised a medical student?

A. About 6 years ago.

This line of questioning reveals the witness's tendency to embellish his or her professional credentials and would probably have a negative impact on the witness's credibility.

When a physician witness is marginally qualified to testify, the opposing lawyer will question the extent or relevance of the witness's experience in the specific medical matter being argued. For example,

- Q. Have you had specialized training with this particular disease?

- Q. You haven't seen very many patients with this problem, have you?

- Q. Isn't it true that patients with this illness aren't usually referred to doctors in your specialty?

The value of expert witnesses is their specialized knowledge that will aid the triers of fact. If the average juror can independently understand the issues in a trial, then an expert witness is not needed. In voir dire the cross-examiner might reduce the expert's input to "common sense" and thus argue to exclude the testimony as unnecessary.

- Q. Doctor, you are here today to testify about the risk factors that underlie low back injuries, is that correct?

- A. Yes.

- Q. You have a list of factors that raise the risk of low back injury, don't you?

- A. Yes, I do.

- Q. One of the elements of daily life that contribute to back problems is poor posture, correct?

- A. Yes, that's right. For example, if you slouch when sitting, you put extra strain on the spine and ligaments.

- Q. Another risk factor is lack of exercise, right?

- A. Yes.

- Q. Another is poor body mechanics—how you bend, lift, push, and twist—isn't that right?

- A. Yes.

- Q. And being overweight is not good for your back, right?

- A. Right.

Q. Is emotional stress also a risk factor?

A. Yes. When the body is under stress, muscles become tighter and shorter, decreasing spinal flexibility and increasing the likelihood of injury.

Q. Is diet also a risk factor?

A. Yes, it is.

Q. These risk factors—poor posture, lack of exercise, stress, and diet—they kind of make sense when you think about it, don't they?

A. Yes, they do.

Q. So, it's common sense to exercise, watch what you eat and so forth, to take care of your back, right?

This is an important question. If you say, "No," you will not be believed. If you say, "Yes," you are admitting that the lay jurors know about the risk factors for low back injury and that your expertise is not needed. It is better to reply:

A. These risk factors make definite sense to a health professional who has training and experience in this field, like myself.

This response reminds the court that these notions are best understood by a person with medical and biological expertise.

When a medicolegal case involves a newly identified syndrome or a novel treatment approach, the opposing counsel may object to the medical testimony on the basis of a Daubert challenge. According to the 1993 ruling by the U.S. Supreme Court on *Daubert v. Merrell Dow Pharmaceuticals*, expert testimony is admissible if it is based on scientific methodology that has been subjected to peer review and accepted by members of the scientific community.[3] Outside the presence of the jury, the judge may ask the physician witness:

Q. Has the theory or technique been tested scientifically?

Q. Has it been subjected to peer review and journal publication?

Q. Is there a known or potential rate of error?

Q. Has it achieved a degree of acceptance within the relevant scientific community?

In these cases the judge must scrutinize very closely the credentials, methodology, and conclusions of the expert to be assured that an appropriately scientific basis exists for the opinions being proffered in court. Thus, if the physician witness can explain that the patient's unusual diagnosis is supported by peer-reviewed professional publications or that the recently developed medical technique has received acceptance by the scientific community, the judge will allow the physician to testify. The Daubert standard is generally considered to be more liberal than the previously held Frye rule that required that the expert witness's opinion be based on *generally accepted* scientific principles.[4]

In the real world, a physician's credentials are rarely challenged. Thus, in court you may feel offended, threatened, defensive, or angered by these apparent attacks on your qualifications. Withhold these natural reactions and try to answer these probing questions patiently and accurately in a conservative demeanor.

Most probably the opposing attorney's testing of your qualifications will not result in your being excluded as an expert witness, but your responses may determine the weight given by the jurors to your testimony. They may, for instance, attribute greater credibility to another physician whose credentials appear to be more impressive or germane to the particular trial.

Direct Examination

After the judge rules that you are competent to testify as an expert medical witness, your lawyer will proceed with the direct examination which should be, in essence, a teaching process. The goal of the direct examination is to educate the jury about the medical facts of the case so that they can render a just decision.

The direct examination will first clarify the expert witness's connection with the case, that is, whether you were the treating physician or a medical consultant asked to examine the patient's records and form opinions specifically for the trial. The jury needs to know the basis of your testimony and the nature of the information you possess that led to the conclusions you have reached.

As mentioned in Chapter 1, if you are appearing only as a fact witness, you will testify as to what you have observed in your evaluation and treatment of the patient. More than likely, if you have sufficient knowledge of the case, you will be testifying as an expert witness and permitted to proffer your opinions on the case, such as the cause of the putative injury or the motivations of the patient.

You will notice that the questions asked in direct examination are open-ended, such as:

Q. Doctor, tell us what you found in your clinical examination of the patient.

Q. What were the findings of the CT scan?

In contrast, closed-ended or leading questions suggest the answer, as in:

Q. The findings of your clinical examination were essentially normal, weren't they?

Q. Did the CT scan show a brain contusion?

Unlike in cross-examinations, attorneys in direct examinations are prohibited from leading the witness because, by asking such a question, the lawyer and not the witness is testifying. Instead, the questioning must allow the witnesses to be independent in stating their findings and conclusions. There is an up-side to open-ended questions. Rather than limiting the witness to yes-or-no answers in a series of closed-ended questions, the open-ended questions provide ample opportunity for the expert to teach the jury about the medical technicalities in the case and are especially effective when the witness is a naturally gifted speaker who can proceed in a narrative form with little or no interruptions. With less eloquent witnesses, the lawyer may prefer to elicit the testimony with a question-by-question approach.[5]

The questioning of a treating physician will include the following typical questions:

Q. Doctor, when was the first time you saw this patient?

Q. Who referred the patient to you?

Q. Tell us what complaints and symptoms the patient presented to you on that first visit.

Q. Describe the physical examination you conducted.

Q. What medical tests did you order?

Q. What were the results of those medical tests?

Q. On the basis of your medical examination and test results, what diagnosis did you reach?

Q. What treatment did you provide that day?

Q. Did you refer the patient for a consultation by a specialist?

Q. Describe the patient's response to your treatment.

Q. Are there going to be long-term effects on the patient's health?

Q. Tell us about any permanent impairment or disability the patient will have.

Q. What kind of future medical care will the patient need?

An experienced attorney will be able to bring out the above pieces of information in a logically organized manner. When you are well prepared and can anticipate the sequence of questions, you may be tempted to answer quickly, even before the question is completely asked. Quick responses could be seen as part of a rehearsed act and should be avoided. On the other hand, taking too much time to answer will make you appear unsure about your conclusions.

For the outside physician witness who has not examined the patient, a different line of questioning is employed. The presenting attorney will ask a *hypothetical question* by setting forth the facts in evidence as well as those expected to be placed in evidence that form the foundation of the opinion and then ask for the expert's opinion. An example, albeit abbreviated, might be

Q. Doctor, I want you to assume that the plaintiff was a healthy person with no previous neck, back, or headache problems, and she slips and falls at the defendant's office, landing on her buttocks and then striking the floor with the back of her head. Assume further that she immediately experiences a sharp pain in her lower back and suffers dizziness and headaches that persist till the present day. Assume that both her personal physician and her orthopedic surgeon have opined that she has a lumbosacral sprain and a cervical strain. Based on these assumed facts, would you agree, with a reasonable degree of medical certainty, that her current neck and back pain are due to the slip and fall accident?

After the nontreating expert has given an opinion based on the hypothetical question, the witness can be asked to explain the basis of the opinion.

While being questioned, you should be prepared to be interrupted by the opposing counsel's objections. These objections are directed at the form in which the question was asked (e.g., a leading question, or a question calling for conclusions outside the witness's field of expertise, or a hypothetical question with assumed "facts" contradicted by the evidence), or at the witness's response to the question (e.g., an unresponsive answer or a speculation). When an objection is made, you should stop talking immediately and wait for the ruling of the judge. Objections are standard courtroom procedures that should not be interpreted as an attack on you or your credibility.

In criminal court, a defendant must be found guilty "beyond a reasonable doubt," which is a standard that requires convincing evidence of culpability. In civil court, where most medical experts testify regarding personal injury or medical negligence, opinions are subject to a less stringent standard that is usually expressed as *a reasonable degree of certainty*. As discussed in Chapter 1, the use of the term "reasonable degree of medical certainty" is problematic for physician witnesses. First of all, there is no clear definition for "reasonable certainty."[6] Some doctors mistakenly think that certainty means "100% sure," which is a level of certitude that is incongruent in medicine. "Reasonable certainty" in civil court refers to "preponderance or 51% of the evidence" or "more likely than not."[7] Attorneys sometimes use the term "reasonable probability," which is better understood by the medical doctor. Before testifying, you may want to discuss the "reasonable certainty" definition with an attorney in your jurisdiction.

Physician witnesses should be able to define the phrase "reasonable medical certainty" because they may be asked about its meaning in court.

Q.　Doctor, you stated that your opinion about the cause of the plaintiff's injuries was based on a reasonable degree of medical certainty, is that correct?

A.　Yes.

Q. Could you explain what is meant by "a reasonable degree of medical certainty"?

A. It means "more likely than not." In other words, the accident was, more likely than not, the cause of the patient's injuries.

If the expert claims not to know the meaning of the phrase "reasonable certainty" or states,

a.* It means I was reasonably sure.

the judge could exclude the witness's entire testimony.[8]

After you express your opinions to a reasonable degree of medical certainty, you will be asked to explain the rationale behind the opinions.

Q. Doctor, please tell the court how you arrived at your conclusions.

This is the time to explain the medical issues involved in the case, such as the physical damages sustained and the clinical findings and test results that support your observations and, of utmost importance in lawsuits, the cause of the injuries.

Most physicians misunderstand the legal definition of *causation* because, from their medical experience, they equate cause with etiology and consider all possible causes of a patient's medical condition. In legal terms, the proximate cause of an injury is a particular event that *precipitates, hastens, or aggravates* an aspect of the patient's medical condition.[9] Thus, if a person is struck by a car, undergoes hip surgery, and suffers a cardiac arrest during the operation, from a legal standpoint in most jurisdictions, the heart attack would be considered to be caused by the traffic accident. Because of the crucial role of causation in any litigation, physicians must understand the medicolegal meaning of causation.

The opinions you express in court must be based on objective and verifiable information.[2] By referring to test results used to arrive at your conclusions and by consistent reference to hard medical evidence, you will be more convincing and receive more acceptance from the court.

---

*Throughout this book, weak and ineffectual answers are preceded by a lowercase "a," whereas better responses are preceded by a capital "A."

You want the jurors to be able to recall in the jury room your concrete findings and the key evidence that supports your conclusions.

During the more technical and complex aspects of the testimony, your answers should be brief and in plain language. It is difficult for the average juror to grasp extended scientific explanations. No matter how comprehensive your medical summarization is, if the jurors are confused or overwhelmed by the information, you will fail to teach them anything about the case. To clarify your points, the use of demonstrative evidence, such as photographs or charts, can be especially effective as an adjunct to the purely verbal explanations.

As the questions about your opinions unfold, it is important to recognize the limits of your area of competence. There may be a fine line between an opinion based on firm empirical findings and one based on conjecture. Do not guess or speculate; you must be reasonably certain in your responses. There is also a fine line between your sphere of expertise (e.g., neurology) and another physician's specialty (e.g., neuroradiology). When the questioning extends into an area that is beyond your knowledge and experience, you should indicate that you do not feel competent to express an opinion. It is perfectly acceptable to say, "I don't know" or "That is beyond my area of expertise." The court will respect professionals who admit to limits in their expertise rather than testifying on matters for which they have inadequate training or experience.[7]

Closing Arguments

This chapter described the qualification process, which is usually a series of routine questions about the witness's educational and professional experiences. Through a voir dire cross-examination, the opposing attorney may try to prevent the physician from offering any testimony, narrow the witness's field of expertise, or at least diminish the weight of the testimony by a probing critique of the witness's medical background. The pitfalls of any attempt to embellish or exaggerate one's credentials in the courtroom are obvious.

More often than not the physician's qualifications are not aggressively challenged and are accepted with little debate. This is particularly true when the doctor is experienced or has clearly impressive professional credentials. In this initial phase of courtroom questioning, the attorneys on both sides are attempting to verify the strengths and limitations of the expert witness. But because physicians' authority outside of the courtroom is usually honored without question by their patients and colleagues, physicians invariably feel offended by these attacks on their professional credentials. It is important to remain calm and not react defensively to these questions about your credentials.

The direct examination, conducted by the attorney who desires your testimony, should proceed relatively smoothly, particularly if you have engaged in some pretrial preparations. If possible, briefly rehearse, but not memorize, your testimony, practicing everyday language to explain your medical opinions. At the trial, through a series of open-ended questions, you will be able to explain your findings so that the jury can understand the major medical issues of the case.

This is just the start of your testifying, and you would be wise to conserve your energy for the critical questions that are likely to be asked in the next phase by the opposing counsel in cross-examination.

References

1. Matson JV. *Effective Expert Witnessing: A Handbook for Technical Professionals*. Chelsea, MI: Lewis Publishers, 1990.
2. Tigar ME. *Examining Witnesses*. Chicago: American Bar Association, 1993.
3. *Daubert v. Merrell Dow Pharmaceuticals*, 113 SCt 2786, 61 LW 4805 (1993).
4. Ayala FJ, Black B. Science and the courts. *Am Sci* 1993;81:230–239.
5. James AE (ed). *Legal Medicine: With Special Reference to Diagnostic Imaging*. Baltimore: Urban & Schwarzenberg, 1980.
6. Rossi FF. *Expert Witnesses*. Chicago: American Bar Association, 1991.
7. Appelbaum PS, Gutheil TG. *Clinical Handbook of Psychiatry and the Law* (2nd ed). Baltimore: Williams & Wilkins, 1991.
8. Babitsky S, Mangraviti JJ Jr. *How to Excel During Cross-Examination: Techniques for Experts that Work*. Falmouth, MA: SEAK, 1997.
9. Danner D, Sagall EL. Medicolegal causation: a source of professional misunderstanding. *Am J Law Med* 1977;3:303–308.

4

Cross-Examination

The cross-examination is an essential part of every trial. The purpose of the cross-examination is to give the opposing attorney an opportunity to challenge the testimony given by a witness during direct examination. The cross-examiner will try to elicit answers that are helpful to the cross-examiner's side of the lawsuit or that discredit the value of the witness's direct testimony.[1] In short, the aim of the cross-examination is to obtain admissions or concessions that are favorable to the opposing side of the case.

Most witnesses are aware of the adversarial nature of a cross-examination and are understandably apprehensive about this phase of testifying. Historically, lawyers were given considerable freedom for dramatics and verbal combativeness, which have become fodder for many classic books, plays, and films. Legal authorities observe that the courts today are intent on maintaining decorum and are less tolerant of lawyer histrionics and harassment, thereby safeguarding witnesses from unnecessary duress while on the witness stand.[2] The rules of court prevent the trial attorney from arguing with the witness or attempting to embarrass the witness. Furthermore, the cross-examining lawyer is not allowed to go far beyond the testimony given during direct examination or to repeat the same question excessively. While expert witnesses need not fear that the opposing attorney will be abusive, they must be prepared for a vigorous questioning designed to diminish the testimony given in direct examination.

It is especially important to transfer the professional demeanor shown during the direct examination into the cross-examination. Keep the same pleasant, businesslike tone you had during the direct examination. There is no need to change to a more severe manner or defensive attitude simply because you are now facing the opposing lawyer. Your professional conduct and confidence during this critical portion of testifying will enhance your credibility with the jury.

During the cross-examination, remain calm and be alert to all questions. Wait for the entire question to be asked and do not give an answer before the lawyer completes the question. Your patience in responding will give the attorney who provided the direct examination a chance to object if the question is vague or is inappropriate in any way. The pause before answering also gives you the time to contemplate the best answer to the question.

As in the direct examination, answer all questions in the cross-examination responsively within the realm of reasonable medical certainty. Do not be an advocate and form your answers to help win the case. The advocates in court are the attorneys on both sides, and it is their responsibility, not yours, to win the case.

Given the adversarial nature of our courtroom system, attorneys feel obliged to attack the expert witness on cross-examination. You must remember that it is part of the lawyer's job to try to discredit the witness, including questioning your credibility and integrity, and it is essential that you do not take the aggressive questioning personally.

In addition, you may find it difficult under intense cross-examination to maintain a posture of neutrality. The impartial, scientific role is desirable, but you must also be prepared to respond to a persistent cross-examination with an equally forceful presentation. Considerable effort and self-discipline are needed to preserve your testimony, remain the objective expert, and demonstrate a balanced judgment and a sense of fair play.

Do not answer questions that are unclear, or if there are words in the questions that are unclear, or if there are words in the questions that need to be better defined. You may say

A. I'm sorry. Could you rephrase the question?

A. I can't answer that question. Can you define "authoritative" for me?

If you do not know the answer to the question, say

A. I don't know.

The jury understands that you cannot know everything in a complex field such as medicine and will appreciate your acknowledging your limitation rather than being an arrogant know-it-all.

While you testify, it is good to be confident about your medical expertise, but it is naive to believe that you are the only one in the courtroom who understands the biological and scientific issues of the case. Unless you are fortunate enough to be involved in an attorney's first case in court, you will probably be cross-examined by the average trial lawyer who specializes in civil tort and has been involved in numerous personal injury litigations. Such an attorney has done considerable reading in the medicolegal sphere in the past and has probably consulted with several medical experts of different specialties. The opposing attorney may even have hired a medical consultant specifically to help formulate an attack on your findings. In short, it is wiser to assume that the cross-examiner is knowledgeable about medicolegal issues in your field and has the ability to engage in very insightful and sophisticated inquiry about the case.[2] If the cross-examiner is indeed inexperienced and inept, be patient and do not be abrupt or patronizing.

On occasion there may be little or no cross-examination. The opposing attorney will choose not to cross-examine an experienced expert witness who appears to be truthful and capable and who has a well-documented set of opinions. More questioning would simply buttress an already convincing direct examination. In this case, the attorney will decide that the best cross-examination is no cross-examination. On other occasions, the opposing counsel may realize that a critical point has been overlooked or omitted in the direct examination and may not want to cross-examine and give the expert witness an added opportunity to submit the important information.[3] Finally, there may be little or no cross-examination if the direct testimony is uncontentious or non-damaging to the other side.

The duty of cross-examining lawyers is to closely examine the evidence, to ensure that the facts were reported accurately, and to probe for alternative interpretations of the facts that would be favorable to their client's case. The physician witness should realize that it is the responsibility of cross-examining attorneys to try to weaken the expert's testimony and to present the possibility of doubt for the sake of their client and in the interests of justice, and that it is not the goal of cross-examination to publicly embarrass the expert witness. Most attorneys cross-examine with due courtesy for the physician witness who is honest, but will become a hostile questioner with the witness who is not.[3] Furthermore, a lawyer's attempt to humiliate a cooperative physician witness will not be appreciated by lay jurors or the judge. Thus, the witness who testifies with candor on solidly based evidence has less to worry about in a cross-examination.

Leading Questions and Hypothetical Questions

To ensure a thorough cross-examination, the courts provide the opposing attorney with greater leeway in asking questions, such as asking leading questions or hypothetical questions.[2] The cross-examiner is also given a wide latitude in asking questions pertaining to the direct examination testimony as well as questions about other testimony in the case. The cross-examination may also include challenging the medical knowledge of the physician witness.

Leading Questions

In a cross-examination, a witness may purposely or subconsciously evade clear interrogation. To avoid evasiveness and ensure a direct answer from an adverse witness, the cross-examiner will ask leading questions. A leading question is one that contains the desired answer within the question itself. For example,

Q. Didn't you see the patient only on two occasions?

Q. You prescribed Relafen, didn't you?

Q. Isn't it true that you considered a psychiatric referral for the patient?

Q. *Internal Medicine,* edited by J.H. Stein, is an authoritative text, is it not?

The leading question is a highly effective tool for the cross-examining attorney who has the opportunity to phrase questions that limit the witness to "Yes" or "No" answers.

Cross-examining lawyers utilize additional techniques to encourage certain answers from the witness. For instance, on occasion, the attorney will shake his or her head from side to side while asking a question, such as

Q. You didn't have time to order all of the tests you needed, did you?

The head shaking would subtly suggest that the answer should be

    A. No.

At other times the attorney will ask a series of three or four consecutive questions in which the obvious answer is "Yes," followed by a question in which the best answer should be "No." However, after a series of "Yes" answers a witness can be lulled into a "Yes" mental set and unintentionally respond "Yes" incorrectly.

Some leading questions are heavily loaded, suggesting that the answer should be "Yes" even though you may believe otherwise. For example,

    Q. Doctor, you would agree, wouldn't you, that the patient could have had more improvement in his condition if he came for his appointments regularly?

You can avoid being misled into answering incorrectly by carefully listening to each question in its entirety and understanding the nature of the leading question. With certain questions you may not want to limit yourself to a simple "Yes" or "No" answer. If you state that a "Yes" or "No" answer is insufficient, you will probably be allowed by the judge to explain your answer more fully. Thus, you can state

    A. I will answer the question and I would like to provide a full explanation of my answer.

You only need to respond to the question that is being asked. Do not worry about all of the ramifications of your answer and, most of all, avoid worrying about winning the argument or winning the case. For instance, to the question

    Q. Is Tegretol a good medication to treat partial complex seizures?

give a simple "Yes" or "No" response. You are not required to give a complete explanation of the purpose of the medication or all of the adverse reactions from taking this medicine. Anticipate follow-up questions such as

    Q. How does Tegretol help the patient's condition?

Q. What are the side effects of taking this medicine?

Answer each of these questions, one at a time, no more and no less.

Hypothetical Questions

One of the more difficult courtroom techniques you will contend with in cross-examination is the hypothetical question.[4] The opposing counsel wants to alter your position and may try to do this by asking you a hypothetical question, incorporating certain factors you may not have considered in reaching your conclusions.

Q. Doctor, I want you to assume the following: that a person slipped and fell in a store, stood up immediately, and continued to shop for another 10 minutes. I want you to further assume that she shopped in the mall for an additional half hour, made a few purchases, and carried two large shopping bags to her car. Finally, I want you to assume that she went home and cooked a meal for her family of four before retiring for the evening, and did not tell anyone that she had any injury or back pain, and did not seek medical help until 10 days later. Doctor, given this description, does it sound like this woman did or did not injure her back from that slip and fall in the store?

A. Given that description, I would say that she probably did not injure her back.

It is tempting to conclude, given those obvious facts, that no injury took place. If the hypothetical question included many or most of the essential factors you need to reach a diagnosis, then you may form an opinion for the jury, or you may say

A. Given those descriptions, I would have to re-evaluate the entire case. At this point I cannot answer your question.

or

A. I need some time to consider your question. I cannot respond immediately.

If the hypothetical factors are irrelevant or insufficient to draw a conclusion with reasonable certainty, the hypothetical question cannot be answered, in which case the following reply should be given:

  A.   Without more information, I cannot render an opinion. (Be prepared to indicate what further information you need to form an opinion.)

Some expert witnesses mistakenly believe that the hypothetical question is purely theoretical and has no bearing on the case. In such instances, the witness might answer very freely and offer contradictory testimony. When the assumptions made in the hypothetical questions are identical to the real situation, the answers given apply to the case at hand. Thus, in the example given above, based on the assumptions provided, if the expert witness stated that the woman probably did not injure her back, then this would be the witness's opinion for the case being tried.

Goals in Cross-Examination

The goals in the cross-examination of a medical expert witness are to demonstrate that

  1.   The physician witness lacks qualifications and credibility.

  2.   The medical evidence is questionable.

  3.   The medical conclusions are questionable.

  4.   There are grounds for impeachment because of contradictory or inconsistent testimony.

  5.   The physician witness is biased.

Lacking Qualifications and Credibility

The cross-examiner will argue for lack of qualifications by demonstrating that the witness has inadequate education or relevant training, lack of clinical practice, absence of board certification, limited experience with the kind of medical case involved in the trial, and other evidence of insufficient knowledge. The professional backgrounds of expert witnesses will be closely scrutinized in order to minimize their credibility. Some of the ways the opposing attorney will try to prove this point are given below.

"Doctor, do you know what you're talking about?"

During the cross-examination, the opposing attorney has the right to test the competency of the expert witness with respect to the scientific issues of the case. Having done some homework on this matter, the attorney might ask some of these penetrating questions:

> Q. What are some of the current controversies pertaining to the diagnosis of _____ disease?
>
> Q. Have you read the article by _____ that appeared in the *Annals of Internal Medicine* earlier this year?
>
> Q. Would you agree with Dr. _____'s theory regarding the etiology of _____ disease?

Answer these questions as honestly and fully as you can. If you are well versed on the topic, this is an opportune time to demonstrate your professional competence to the jury and judge. However, you are not expected to have read every prominent article or author on a specific medical topic, and you can say

> A. No, I have not read that particular article. I would be glad to review that article if you wish.

The way to prevent any embarrassment along these lines is to review your own textbooks and testify that there are several authorities in the field.

> A. I am not familiar with Dr. _____'s theory, but I have read the works of Dr. _____ and Dr. _____ regarding this disease. Would you like me to tell you what they've said?

"You mean you're not a board-certified doctor?"

A physician's credibility may also be challenged if the witness is not board certified.

> Q. Could you tell the jury what it means to be board certified by the American Board of Internal Medicine?

A. Board certification by the American Board of Internal Medicine means that a physician graduates from an accredited medical school, successfully completes an approved residency in internal medicine, and passes the examination established by the American Board of Internal Medicine.

Q. Doctor, are you board certified by the American Board of Internal Medicine?

A. No, I'm not.

Q. Are you board certified by any board?

A. No.

Q. Why not?

a. Well, I don't need a board certification. I'm licensed by this state to practice medicine, and I participate in continuing medical education to retain my active license. Years ago I thought about getting my board certifications but it's a very time-consuming process and I've been too busy treating patients and keeping my practice going to prepare for those tests. Maybe one of these days I'll go through the trouble of getting my boards. You know you have to travel out of state to complete the process.

This long and involved answer is unnecessarily detailed and sounds overly defensive. A briefer factual response is preferred.

A. Board certification is not needed for a physician to practice medicine.

A better response is to emphasize your experience and area of competence.

A. I am not board certified, but I have completed approved postgraduate training and have over 10 years of experience in treating the disorder we are discussing today.

"You're really not sure, are you?"

There will be times when your credibility is questioned because you hesitate longer than usual before answering a question. The attorney will pick up on this and ask

Q. Doctor, you are not sure of your answer, are you?

a. I guess so.

Q. It's been a long time since your examination of the patient, so you're not sure about what you observed, right?

a. That's right.

The witness who admits to being unsure may have some or all of the testimony disregarded. Do not allow the attorney to undermine your confidence and your testimony. Stand by your conclusions and do not let the lawyer change your testimony. Instead, reply

A. I have not seen the patient for some time, but I have her records to rely on. I hesitated in answering your last question because I wanted to be certain about my answer.

"Doctor, where is the medial longitudinal fasciculus, or MLF, located?"

In an attempt to highlight the fallibility of a physician witness, some attorneys employ an age-old tactic of asking you to define obscure anatomic terminology that you have not heard of since medical school. You need to know the subject matter about which you are testifying, but you are not expected to know everything about medicine, and you need not hesitate to say

A. I don't know. That does not come up in my specialty practice of pediatric medicine.

The response emphasizes that you are a pediatric specialist, a fact which is most relevant to the case.

A. I don't know, but I can find the answer for you if it is important to this case.

This answer stresses that the question may not be pertinent at all to the case and unveils the attorney's futile attempt to discredit the witness.

Questionable Medical Evidence

The opposing attorney can hinder the expert witness's testimony by challenging the data on which the medical conclusions are reached. The aim here is to show that the evidence obtained is based on an inadequate examination or on incomplete or incorrect information.

"Is that all the information you had?"

To question the bases of an expert witness's opinion, the opposing attorney will ask questions such as:

Q. Didn't you rely heavily on just an x-ray?

Q. Weren't there other tests you could have ordered to confirm your findings?

Q. Wouldn't it be better to have had the medical records of the previous treating physicians?

Do not overreact to these valid queries about your data base. Avoid defensive answers such as:

a. Of course I relied on the x-ray. I trust the results of those tests.

a. Sure, I could have ordered more tests. But they cost money and in these days of managed care we have to be cost-conscious.

a. No, I had a thorough examination of the patient and I didn't need any previous records. Besides, those patient records are always hard to read.

You would do better to offer more carefully thought-out answers.

A. I relied on many sources for my diagnosis, including the x-rays, my clinical examination, and the various other tests I ordered.

A. More data are always helpful, but I believe I had sufficient medical information to reach a reliable diagnosis.

**"Are you telling me that you based your
diagnosis only on what the patient told you?"**

Many medical diagnoses are reached on the basis of information
obtained from the patient. Physicians have been trained to formulate
diagnostic impressions relying on the patient's symptoms and recollec-
tions, whereas the average layperson may expect that extensive and
expensive test results are mandatory to make a diagnosis. Thus, the following questions may be asked in cross-examination:

Q. Besides taking the history of his condition from the patient,
   what tests did you order?

A. I didn't order any tests.

Q. Not even a blood or urine test?

A. No.

Q. Why not?

A. Because with this condition, there are no tests that will detect the illness. I rely on the history the patient gives me to make the diagnosis.

Q. You mean you based your diagnosis just on what the man told you?

a. Yes.

The "Yes" answer, though accurate, may be insufficient. The jury needs
to hear the reasons why your conclusions were reached without medical tests being done.

A. The patient told me that he had a strong family history of
   migraine and a pattern of vascular headaches since his teens, as
   well as an aura followed by scintillating scotoma and a throb-
   bing unilateral headache. The pattern of symptoms, in addition
   to his clinical appearance in my office, made it quite clear to
   me that he has vascular headaches. I did not need to order further tests to come to the diagnosis of classical migraine.

"Would you change your opinion if . . . ?"

Because your opinion is based on certain factors, the opposing attorney will test your opinion by offering other information you may not
have considered.

Q. Would you change your opinion if you were aware that the patient had a second accident after you treated him?

a. No, I would stick to my original conclusions.

The above answer is an untenable position and should not be considered.

a. Yes, I probably would have to change my opinion.

As can be seen, this form of questioning can be difficult to answer. If you say, "No," you may appear close-minded to facts that are relevant. On the other hand, a "Yes" answer could negate all of your proffered opinions. A better response would be

A. I would like to know more about the second accident before I offer any additional opinions. I would also like to re-examine the patient in light of this new information.

"What do you mean, 'You don't know . . . ,' Doctor?"

When you do not have all of the information about a patient's medical background, it is best to admit it by stating, "I don't know." The opposing attorney may want to amplify your lack of knowledge and proceed to ask several similar questions to elicit more "I don't know" answers in an effort to fluster you and cause you to blurt out impulsive and poorly thought-out statements.[2]

Q. Do you know which doctors previously treated your patient?

A. No.

Q. Then you don't know what they found, do you?

A. No.

Q. And you have no idea what treatments or medicines were prescribed to your patient, right?

a. Yes, it's true that I don't know who his previous doctors were, or what they found, or what treatment or medicines were prescribed. You're just trying to show that I don't know anything, but you're wrong. I know a lot about this patient. You just haven't asked the right questions.

A blatantly defensive answer such as this does little to help your image as a competent physician. Your best answer is to admit your lack of knowledge and reply

A. It's true that I don't know some aspects of the patient's previous medical treatment, but I am aware of the various findings I obtained that clearly indicated the nature of his present condition.

Questionable Medical Conclusions

The expert witness's conclusions can be the most damaging to an opposing lawyer's case. Thus, cross-examination will surely entail attacks on the reasoning behind the expert's opinion, such as the following:

"Can an injured man play basketball?"
On occasion the attorney will challenge the expert's conclusions by identifying certain events that are inconsistent with the doctor's diagnosis.

Q. Doctor, were you aware that the day after he allegedly injured his hand at work, your patient played a full game of basketball for his church's team?

A. No. I wasn't aware of that.

Q. Given the fact that he played basketball after the supposed work injury, isn't it possible he actually injured his hand some time afterward, say, playing basketball on his own time?

a. Yes, that's possible.

Indeed there is a likelihood that the patient's hand injury occurred outside the workplace, but the fact that he played basketball may not be sufficient to contradict the testimony. A fairer answer might be

A. I don't know anything about the basketball game. I don't know if he had any pain or if he favored his injured hand during the game. I do know that he reported his hand injury immediately at the work site, and he was seen by the infirmary nurse who felt that an orthopedic consultation was in order.

"Medicine is more an art than a science, right?"

A frequent line of argument is to attack medicine and medical diagnoses as being unscientific. While there are indeed many scientific aspects of medicine, physicians are aware that much is unknown about many areas of medical practice.

Q. When you look at all the medical findings you have on a patient, is there a scientific formula or technical manual you follow that tells you exactly what the diagnosis is?

A. No.

Q. Isn't it true that the process of synthesizing all the medical data to reach a diagnosis—that's a skill you develop over the years, isn't that right?

A. That's right.

Q. Then, wouldn't you agree that the practice of medicine is more of an art than a science, like nuclear physics?

a. I'd agree.

The acceptance of medicine as an art will probably weaken this witness's testimony in the eyes of the jury, who expect to be relying on scientific expertise. A better reply would be

A. Medicine is not nuclear physics, but medicine is based on scientific theory and research. The opinions I offer today are rooted in medical science.

Another attack on medicine as science may be seen in questions about the future.

Q. If medicine is a science, can you tell us if the chance of this patient recovering is 50%, 75%, or 99%?

a. No, I can't give such exact percentages.

An expert witness is not obligated to give exact predictions in terms of percentages.[4] Expert witnesses express their opinions in terms of reasonable medical certainty, which is 51% likelihood, and can reply

    A. I cannot give you an exact percentage, but I can tell you that it is more likely than not that he will recover from these injuries so that he can return to his usual line of work.

A physician need not be defensive about the state of the medical sciences. Attacks on the limits of medicine as a science can provide an opportunity for the witness to educate the jury on current findings and developments.

    A. Progress in medical science is constantly advancing, which is why physicians are required to obtain continued education to keep us abreast of our medical specialties.

"But, doesn't your opinion conflict with that of Dr. DeBakey?"

The courtroom adversary system invariably leads to the presentation of opposing medical opinions in what is often referred to as "the battle of the experts." Attorneys will challenge an expert witness's conclusions by bringing forth the conflicting findings of other medical experts such as:

    Q. Your diagnosis differs with the diagnosis made by the pathologist, right?

    Q. Isn't it true that three other medical doctors came to the same conclusion that differs from yours?

    Q. Wouldn't you defer to Dr. _____, who has had the opportunity to review far more medical records of this patient than you have?

An expert witness who is less than confident may blurt out damaging answers, such as:

    a. Well, I'm the attending physician and I make the diagnosis, not the pathologist.

a. I don't care if 30 doctors differ with me. I know what I found and I'm confident I'm right.

a. Well, Dr. _____ is a well-known expert. I wouldn't hesitate to defer to her.

Rather than the above, consider these more thoughtful responses:

A. I appreciated the report by the pathologist. However, I had considerably more data available to me as the attending doctor, and my conclusions are based on the totality of solid medical evidence.

A. I am not sure why those three physicians reached opinions that differ from mine. It is possible for reasonable differences to occur among doctors. I am certain that my conclusions are based on well-substantiated diagnostic information.

A. No, I need not defer to anyone on this matter. As I have stated before, my conclusions are based on well-substantiated medical evidence.

A physician witness need not be alarmed or defensive when differing opinions are presented in a case. Other acceptable responses are

A. Medical cases are sometimes open to debate. I have offered you my opinion and the other doctor gave a different opinion. We do not agree on this case.

A. We don't always agree at the hospital. I'm not surprised that there is a disagreement here in court.

Physicians regularly disagree at staff meetings and at professional conferences; there is no reason why they should not have different opinions in the courtroom. How you react to the opposing expert's testimony is critical. Clearly you want to avoid rude put-downs such as "That's idiotic!" or "That's a lot of bull." If a different approach or school of thought is presented, it is a mistake to reject it outright, for example, "They don't know what they're talking about." What you believe is an expression of confidence is seen as a show of arrogance, which does not go over well with jurors. Take the high road and acknowledge reasonable differences among professionals, while asserting your own firm position.

"Don't normal people feel the same way as your patient?"

A frequently used technique to challenge diagnoses is to focus on separate symptoms and to relate them to everyday health problems.

> Q. Doctor, you referred to your patient as having abdominal distress, didn't you?
>
> A. Yes, I did.
>
> Q. Abdominal distress—is that like a belly ache?
>
> A. Yes.
>
> Q. Normal healthy people have abdominal distress, don't they?
>
> A. Yes, they do.
>
> Q. You said that she has migraines. That's bad headaches, right?
>
> A. Right.
>
> Q. Normal healthy people have bad headaches, don't they?
>
> A. Yes.
>
> Q. And she has had diarrhea, right?
>
> A. Yes.
>
> Q. We all have experienced that, haven't we?
>
> a. I think so.

The attorney's effort to minimize the patient's symptoms is fairly transparent. Without any comment from the medical witness, the jury might conclude that the patient only had normal everyday health problems. Hence, the medical witness needs to remind the court that symptoms taken separately have no clinical significance and that physicians reach diagnoses by considering the entire pattern of symptoms presented by the patient.

> A. By itself, diarrhea is a common everyday problem that may not be serious. However, when the patient presented with severe headaches, stomach pain, and diarrhea, I suspected that she might have influenza, and the tests I ordered confirmed my suspicions.

Inconsistent Testimony

An expert witness's testimony may be impeached by showing that the doctor has on previous occasions made statements inconsistent with the present testimony. When these statements are in written reports or in pretrial depositions, these documents will be offered as evidence that could be sufficient to impeach the expert's entire testimony.

"But you said in the deposition . . . "

The pretrial deposition taken at the expert witness's office is a sworn testimony. If the physician changes an answer at trial in any way, the deviation from the deposition will immediately be brought to light. For example,

> **Q.** Doctor, your response today in the courtroom is different than it was at your deposition, isn't it true?
>
> **A.** Yes. Since the deposition, I have seen the patient two more times, and there are changes in his condition that led me to change my opinion about his injury.

Matson[5] warns that cross-examiners sometimes take the physician's deposition answer out of context to try to show that the witness is inconsistent with previous testimony.

> **Q.** But, Doctor, you testified in your deposition, on page 18, and I quote "The medicine can cause dangerous side effects." Now you're saying that it doesn't. Which is true, Doctor?

The expert witness always has the right to see the deposition transcript and to review the testimony given earlier. The judge will have a transcript of the deposition made available, and in reviewing it, the witness may discover that the attorney excluded some important information that explains the differences in the answers.

> **A.** The quote you made was incomplete. What I said in the deposition was, "If the patient drank alcohol prior to taking the medicine, the medicine can cause dangerous side effects."

The key point here is to request to review the deposition transcript. Take your time reading the passages carefully so that you can explain why your answer in court differs from your answer in the deposition.

Another technique by the cross-examiner to elicit inconsistent testimony is to repeat the same question, with slight rephrasing. For example, questions such as the following could be asked at different times, in hope of ensnaring the witness if different answers are given:

Q. Will his knee pain interfere with his walking?

Q. So, given the patient's injuries, what are the prospects of his walking normally in the future?

Q. What limitations will his leg injury have in the long run?

Additional variations of these questions could be asked a few more times, and your answer, of course, should be essentially the same. If not, you will appear inconsistent and unreliable, placing your entire testimony in jeopardy.

To help you, objections by the other attorney can be made (e.g., "That question has been asked and answered."). Moreover, you may answer by pointing out

A. As I have testified earlier . . .

A. You asked me the same question earlier, and I said . . .

A. I believe this is the third time you have asked me about the prognosis of his walking. I again say . . .

Biased Witness

When a qualified physician produces testimony based on firm medical evidence and reasoning, the opposing attorney may have little recourse but to focus on possible biases on the part of the expert witness. Note the following tactics:

"So, you admit that you and the attorney have rehearsed the answers you're giving today?"

The cross-examining lawyer may begin the inquiry with a tricky question:

Q. Doctor, have you talked to anyone about this case?

a. No. I haven't.

Your initial reaction might be to say "No" because of the confidential nature of your medical work, perhaps more so in medicolegal cases. A "No" answer would be untrue if you have had any discussion, even a telephone call, with the patient's attorney. In this event, the correct reply is

A. Yes. I have had brief conversations with the patient's attorney, who asked for my opinions about the case.

This is a perfectly acceptable response because it is expected that an expert witness is briefed by an attorney before testifying. Be prepared to be asked about the dates and even the content of the discussions you had with the attorney. A good reply is

A. Yes. I spoke with the patient's attorney, who urged me to answer truthfully, to the best of my ability.

During the cross-examination, the opposing counsel will attempt to discredit the witness by implying that, in pretrial preparations, questions and answers have been thoroughly discussed and planned by the witness and the other attorney, and that the witness is merely a mouthpiece for the attorney.

Q. Doctor, before coming to court, did you have an opportunity to meet with the patient's attorney?

A. Yes, I did.

Q. On how many occasions did you meet with him?

A. We met two times in my office.

Q. And what did you discuss with the attorney?

A. We discussed the upcoming trial and what I was going to say today. I explained the medical issues involved and how this could be clearly presented to the jury.

Q. Did the two of you go over anticipated questions I might be asking?

A. Yes.

Q. And did the two of you discuss how you should respond to my questions?

a. Yes, we did.

Q. So, isn't it fair to say that you and the attorney have rehearsed the answers you're giving today?

a. You could say that.

Agreeing with the last two questions suggests that the witness's answers do not represent the physician's true opinions but are simply answers favoring the plaintiff's side. It is appropriate in pretrial preparations to discuss potential questions, but the answers must only be those of the witness and not influenced by the attorney.

Q. And did the two of you discuss how you should respond to my questions?

A. The attorney told me what questions to expect from you and I told the attorney how I would answer your questions.

Q. Isn't it fair to say that you and the attorney have rehearsed the answers you're giving today?

A. No. The answers I give are mine and mine alone.

How much are you being paid for your opinion today?"

The cross-examining attorney may attempt to impugn your objectivity by implying that you are charging handsome fees and are biased to testify in favor of the side paying you for your expertise. Expect the following kinds of questions:

Q. Doctor, you're being paid to be here today, aren't you?

A. Yes.

Q. How much are you being paid for your testimony?

a. Five hundred dollars an hour.

Expert witnesses are not being paid for their testimony. Otherwise, they are indeed hired guns who are in court merely to mouth the opinions favored by the side who employs them. The appropriate response is

A. I am not being paid for my testimony. I am being paid for my expertise based on the time I spend on this case.

Q. All right then, how much are you being paid for your expertise, Doctor?

A. Five hundred dollars an hour.

Q. And how much time have you spent on this case?

A. I spent two hours examining the patient, and about four hours reviewing her past medical records, and two hours working on my report. All told, about eight hours.

Q. You mean you are being paid four thousand dollars just for telling us that she injured her arm?

A. Yes.

The attempt here by the cross-examiner is to suggest that you are a high-priced mercenary, and it would be normal for you to feel offended and resentful of the implications. Remain calm and professional. Do not succumb to the level of cheap shots and subtle mudslinging being done by the attorney.

Opposing attorneys will also try to advance negative implications if the expert witness's hourly fee for testifying is substantially higher than what is charged for an office visit, if there is a high frequency of prior work with the same attorney or firm, or if the medical witness derives a majority of income from legal activity.

Trying to Upset the Witness

**"You have a reputation of making
this kind of mistake, don't you?"**
The cross-examination can be an intense experience, especially when the opposing lawyer purposely tries to antagonize the witness, hoping to trigger an emotional outburst that would hinder the testimony or would show possible witness bias. Matson[5] provided several examples of inflammatory questions likely to arouse the emotions of even the calmest expert witness, such as:

Q. Doctor, you mean that after all the time and energy you spent on this case, you totally overlooked this critical piece of evidence?

Q. Doctor, couldn't it be that you are just plain wrong in your opinion?

Q. Are you claiming that your opinion is correct and all the other distinguished experts in your field are wrong?

Q. You admit making a mistake. Can you tell us how many more mistakes you made in this case?

Q. If you're not sure, are you saying you don't know what you're talking about?

Q. Haven't you ever been wrong in the past?

With these *ad hominem* questions, it is very difficult to maintain your composure. Remember that if you show your aggravation, you will simply be playing into the opposing lawyer's hands. You will not only lose some credibility, but you may say things that you will regret or that you cannot support with facts. If the lawyer is discourteous while you remain calm and nonargumentative, the jury will resent the lawyer and sympathize with you. Finally, keep in mind that if the lawyer is focusing on issues of bias and fees, this could signal that your credentials and medical opinions are on solid ground and that the only remaining strategy left for the opposing counsel is a personal attack on you. Knowing this might help you feel more confident and less defensive.

Opposing lawyers can also badger physician witnesses by insisting on a "Yes" or "No" answer.[6] Note the following:

Q. Doctor, you stated in your report that it is difficult to reach a clear-cut diagnosis with this patient, isn't that true?

A. That's true, but what I meant was . . .

Q. Doctor, did you or didn't you make that statement?

A. I did, but . . .

Q. This is a simple question, Doctor. Just answer "Yes" or "No."

When you believe that the question cannot be answered with a simple "Yes" or "No," you should say so.

A. I'm sorry. I cannot answer your question with a "Yes" or "No." I would like to explain why.

If it appears that the question cannot be adequately answered with a "Yes" or "No," the judge will permit the witness to answer more fully.

As mentioned before, you must remain calm and not be antagonistic, such as:

   a.   How can I answer if you keep interrupting me? Am I here to testify or not? Are you interested in the whole truth, or just what you want to hear?

An outburst such as this will earn no approval from the jury but a reprimand from the judge, and should be avoided altogether.

In the event that a witness is stubbornly refusing to answer in "Yes" or "No" terms simply to avoid a challenging question, the lawyer can get the judge to order the witness to answer the question. Thus, a witness can, under these circumstances, be compelled to answer "Yes" or "No."

When You Encounter Difficulty

As can be seen by the various challenges and tactics by an opposing attorney, aggressive cross-examination will readily bring on difficulties for an expert witness. The cross-examining lawyer may be exposing a mistake or oversight you made, questioning you in areas in which you are unsure, or exploring a possible contradiction in your testimony. The attorney who has retained you, presumably experienced in court work, can sense that you are in trouble and come to your aid, usually in the form of objections.

Whenever there are objections raised by the attorney, whether in direct or cross-examination, immediately stop talking and wait for a ruling ("sustained" or "overruled") by the judge on the objection. You are not permitted to participate in the discussion on the merits of the objection, even if you have potentially worthwhile input. If the objection is sustained, you are not to answer the question; if it is overruled, you must answer the question.

There are several purposes for an attorney's objection during the cross-examination:

   1.   The attorney who has retained you may be objecting on legal grounds, viz., if the question lacks foundation, or is ambiguous, or is repetitive, or is beyond the scope of your expertise. When the objection is considered valid, the judge will sustain the objection and you need not answer the question. But when the objection is not considered legitimate, the judge will overrule the objection and you must answer the question.

2. In the event you are unaware of the dangerous waters you are treading, the attorney's objection is a kind of wake-up call to make you more conscious of the importance of the questioning you are now facing.

3. The attorney's objections give you some time to consider your answer carefully. The attorney's motivation is particularly apparent when the objections are being overruled by the judge.[5]

The expert witness dealing with a difficult phase of cross-examination can cope in different ways with responses such as:

A. Can you repeat the question?

A. I'm sorry. I don't understand the question.

A. Could you please rephrase the question?

A. The question is too general. Can you be more specific?

A. Can you define _____ ?

A. I can't answer that question without more information.

The point here is to ask the cross-examining attorney to make the question crystal clear, to make sure that you fully understand the question and its ramifications, and to give you valuable additional time to contemplate your best answer. Do not overuse this approach. The aim is not to be evasive or uncooperative, which would negatively impress the jury and judge.

At the End . . .

When the cross-examination ends, there may be a redirect examination to offset any misleading emphasis, ambiguities, or modifications caused by the cross-examination, followed by a recross-examination, and so forth until both sides are satisfied that their questions have been asked and answered. Sometimes, after a witness has completed testifying, an attorney may request the physician to remain in the courthouse in case additional questions come up. If this is inconvenient, you should explain to the judge your important commitments and ask that your examination be completed immediately. The judge will probably grant such a request.[6]

The judge will dismiss you as a witness, and you may then leave the witness stand. Do not spoil your court appearance with a poor exit, such as sighing outwardly in relief. Nor is a broad grin appropriate. Do not smile or wink at the attorney or flash a "thumbs up" or victory sign. These are not indications of an objective or impartial witness. Walk out as you came in, with a confident posture and a businesslike expression, perhaps acknowledging the judge and jury with a nod as you leave.

Closing Arguments

The testimony that emerges during cross-examination may have a greater impact on the jury than the evidence developed during the direct examination. The rigorous questioning from an adverse attorney will alert the jury to listen carefully to the expert's answers and will challenge the expert witness to be as articulate and persuasive as possible. Consequently, it is imperative for you to be prepared for the varied strategies and tactics of an experienced cross-examining attorney, as outlined in this chapter.

The apprehension that you experience before cross-examination is shared by the opposing attorney, who is trained to respect the truthful and capable medical expert witness. Thus, when you are confident in your presentation of the scientific evidence and can justify your medical opinions, the skillful trial lawyer will cross-examine you in a more limited manner, or decide that the best cross-examination is no cross-examination.

When you are on the witness stand, you must understand that a trial is an adversarial procedure and anticipate a grueling cross-examination by the opposing counsel. As Judge Carmi stated, "There is nothing more pitiful than to see a distinguished expert collapse under cross-examination because he or she is ill-prepared or misunderstood the nature of the proceedings."[7]

As opposing attorneys begin to attack your competence and credibility, remember that they are merely doing their job, that is, to weaken the impact of your testimony and to advance their case. Do not take the aggressive questioning personally and do not react with trepidation or with anger. You can remain calm by realizing that you are the medical expert who knows the field better than others in the courtroom, and that you are on the witness stand to share the knowledge you have regarding the medical issues of the case.

References

1. James AE (ed). *Legal Medicine: With Special Reference to Diagnostic Imaging.* Baltimore: Urban & Schwarzenberg, 1980.
2. Liebenson HA. *You, the Expert Witness.* Mundelein, IL: Callaghan & Company, 1962.
3. Gee DJ, Mason JK. *The Courts and the Doctor.* Oxford, England: Oxford University Press, 1990.
4. Shapiro DL. *Psychological Evaluation and Expert Testimony: A Practical Guide to Forensic Work.* New York: Van Nostrand Reinhold, 1984.
5. Matson JV. *Effective Expert Witnessing: A Handbook for Technical Professionals.* Chelsea, MI: Lewis Publishers, 1990.
6. Babitsky S, Mangraviti JJ Jr. *How to Excel During Cross-Examination: Techniques for Experts that Work.* Falmouth, MA: SEAK, 1997.
7. Carmi A. The expert witness in personal injury cases. *Trauma* 1989; 30:5–14.

5

Trial and Error

Ten Ways to Ruin Your Testimony

If you learn best through errors, this is a very educational chapter. Expert witnesses often become their own worst adversary when they self-destruct on the witness stand with thoughtless responses. The following are prime examples of how you can undermine your own testimony in the courtroom:

1. Volunteering unnecessary information
2. Not paying attention to each question
3. Refusing to say, "I don't know"
4. Going beyond your expertise
5. Trying to win the case
6. Being defensive
7. Being disagreeable
8. Accepting authority of books and other witnesses
9. Changing your opinion
10. Letting down your guard

Volunteering Unnecessary Information

"Tell us all you can about the patient."
The medical witness must listen to each question carefully and then provide a responsive but succinct answer.[1,2] Some physicians cannot resist the opportunity to flaunt their medical knowledge; some are simply loquacious. In either case, the witness who fails to give simple and concise answers is giving the opposing attorney opportunities for aggressive questioning. This may especially occur when open-ended questions, like the following, are asked:

Q. What did you do when you conducted your medical examination of the patient?

a. Well, I took a complete history from the child's mother, performed a physical examination, and ordered blood tests. I did not ask for an electrocardiogram or a echocardiogram. I also did not see the need to refer to a pediatric cardiologist.

The witness was asked what was done in the examination of the patient, but was not asked what was *not* done. The additional information simply hands over to the cross-examiner more chances for critical questions, such as:

Q. Why didn't you ask for an electrocardiogram?

Q. Didn't your failure to obtain an echocardiogram preclude your having a complete picture of the patient's condition?

Q. Wouldn't the additional information affect your opinion?

There are many ways in which a witness can fail to limit the answer to the specific facts being asked. Note the following examples:

Q. Doctor, when did you first see the patient?

a. My records show that it was November 13 of last year. I remember it clearly. It was a hectic day, but we were able to squeeze her into my schedule.

(Comment: It would have been sufficient to give the date of the first visit. The additional information contributes nothing, but implies that there may have not been enough time to con-

duct a thorough examination, and the physician now has to ward off accusations about a possibly hurried and inaccurate evaluation. This would be especially damaging if the witness is the defendant in a medical malpractice case.)

Q. Did he show evidence of electrical burns?

a. Now, I don't see too many of these kinds of cases, but this was definitely a case of electrical burns.

(Comment: A simple "Yes" answer is best. The fact that the physician does not see many electrical burns is not essential; the fact that he or she was sure about the diagnosis is.)

Q. What was the cause of the fainting?

a. The fainting was caused by the patient's seizure disorder. I ruled out postural hypotension, diabetes, drug reactions, and any other metabolic problem.

(Comment: The opposing lawyer may, in fact, ask the expert to rule out other causes, but the witness has no obligation to comment on all the possible causes of fainting. The added information, for some jurors, may only serve to muddle an otherwise straightforward situation.)

To be sure, the medical witness has a duty to answer all questions accurately and truthfully, and it is not recommended that the witness withhold essential information called for by the question. The advice here is to be terse and to the point and to avoid rambling. An exception to this rule could be the highly experienced expert witness who can give an impressive mini-lecture to fortify the testimony, although if seen as excessive, arrogant, or pedantic, it can lead to a reprimand from the judge. The inexperienced witness or one who is not a gifted speaker should avoid this tactic.

Not Paying Attention to Each Question

This is obvious: If you don't hear the question, you will give the wrong answer. Opposing lawyers thrive on witnesses giving careless, incorrect responses, and one way that they can entice such answers is to ask a series of consecutive questions for which the correct answer is "Yes," followed by a question for which the answer should be "No."[3–5] The witness who does not pay close attention to each question can be lulled into a "Yes" mind-set and will be highly susceptible to offering an incorrect "Yes" answer, as in this example:

Q. Doctor, you ordered several tests but you didn't ask for an MRI, did you?

A. That's right.

Q. And you didn't request any nuclear diagnostic studies, right?

A. Yes.

Q. Am I correct that you didn't have the records from the City Hospital?

A. Yes.

Q. Nor did you have the records from his personal physician?

A. Yes.

Q. Nor did you have the records from the insurance company?

A. Yes.

Q. So, you didn't have the records from several important sources, right?

a. Yes.

The "Yes" answer is correct if the doctor is truly lacking "records from several important sources." Otherwise, the witness has been duped into giving a wrong and potentially damaging answer, which is now part of the sworn testimony. This occurs when the witness is tired, bored, or distracted with other thoughts. To later change your response or admit that you did not understand the question does not undo the damage. The best prevention for this trap is alertness and careful attention to each question, allowing some time to think about the correct answer.

Refusing to Say "I Don't Know"

"Is there anything you don't know, Doctor?"
Physicians sometimes present themselves as omniscient. These doctors try to answer every question posed to them, regardless of whether they

have adequate knowledge or not.[1,3,4] Being knowledgeable is appreciated by the jury; being a know-it-all is not. Consider this example:

Q. Doctor, you treated this woman when she was hospitalized following her exposure to malathion, is that correct?

A. Yes.

Q. Do you know how long she was exposed to malathion?

A. She told me it was for an hour or so.

Q. Do you know for a fact that it was an hour or so?

a. That's what she told me. It was quite an incident that affected a few other people, too.

Q. Doctor, were you able to verify with any witnesses how long your patient was exposed to malathion?

a. I don't interview witnesses. That's what an investigator does. I'm a doctor and I treat patients.

Q. Are you aware of the specific actions of malathion on the central nervous system?

a. Well, it's a pesticide and an organophosphate, so it's very toxic to our systems and is bound to affect a person in many ways. It's like sniffing glue or breathing gas fumes, but worse.

Q. But do you know how malathion interacts with the brain?

a. Well, I'm not a toxicologist or neurologist, but any physician knows that exposure to a toxic agent like malathion can have many adverse reactions, like dizziness, nausea, and confused thinking.

Q. What published studies are you aware of pertaining to the effects of malathion?

a. There are a number of studies, I'm sure. We've known about the effects of organophosphates for years. At first we didn't realize how it can affect our nervous system, but there have been several reports over the years.

Q. Can you identify any article on this topic?

a. Not offhand. But I probably can find something in my office. I'm sure OSHA can give you some literature, too.

This physician witness's answers are nonresponsive and simply waste valuable courtroom time, a fact not easily forgiven by the jury and judge. For several of the above questions, the witness should in all candor admit to ignorance and realize that certain pieces of information are simply not known by many clinicians. Expert witnesses who are more truthful about their finite knowledge and who are willing to say, "I don't know," will be appreciated by the triers of fact for their honesty and humility.

Going Beyond Your Expertise

"Can you tell us, Doctor, the meaning of life?"
On occasion, attorneys on either side may want you to provide favorable testimony in areas that exceed the range of your expertise.[5,6] As a medical expert you want to be aware of this tactic and clearly demarcate the limits of your competence. You are expected to have general basic knowledge of the medical field, but if the questioning asks for details requiring special knowledge and experience, you should indicate that you do not feel competent to answer the question. Those who go beyond the scope of their competence are likely to face challenges, such as the following:

Q. As a pediatrician, you have testified that this young boy has suffered epileptic seizures for several years, is that correct?

A. Yes.

Q. And these epileptic seizures have led to brain damage and learning problems, correct?

A. Yes.

Q. Now, with his brain damage and learning problems, do you expect him to go to college?

a. No. From what I can tell, he will always have a learning disability and will not be able to go to college.

By answering the last question, the doctor has probably overstepped the boundaries of a pediatrician's expertise. A general pediatrician is not a child psychiatrist or clinical psychologist who has the training and experience to offer a prognosis on this matter. Unless you are a pediatrician with special interests in developmental disorders and educational consultations, you should refrain from offering an opinion, but instead reply

A. I am a pediatrician and cannot answer your question. I would defer to a pediatric neurologist or child psychiatrist as to the future of this boy's education.

The responses given earlier could lead to follow-up questions that could seriously undermine the pediatrician's entire testimony. Note the following:

Q. Doctor, you stated that the boy has a learning disability. What specific kind of learning disability does he have?

A. I don't understand the question.

Q. Well, does he have dyslexia, or a visual perceptual disorder, or a sequencing problem?

A. I don't know specifically what kind of learning disability he has.

Q. Would a pediatric neurologist be familiar with the specific kind of learning disability he has?

A. Probably.

Q. You're not a pediatric neurologist, are you?

A. No. I'm not.

Q. Would a child psychiatrist or a clinical psychologist be familiar with the specific kind of learning disability he has?

A. Yes. I believe so.

Q. You're not trained as a child psychiatrist or clinical psychologist, are you?

A. No. I'm not.

Q. So, you're not trained in the areas of learning disability and special education, correct?

A. That's right.

Q. Doctor, you're in no position to predict that he can't go to college someday, are you?

A.   No. I'm not.

This medical expert may have had important contributions to this trial, such as documenting the patient's seizure disorder, brain damage, and school adjustment problems. However, when you go beyond the boundaries of your competence with bold predictions of a child's future in education, you place your credibility in jeopardy.

Trying to Win the Case

"Are you sure that the sole cause of his depression was his birth trauma?"

Physicians characteristically are patient advocates. They care for their patients and attend to their needs—physical, emotional, and, at times, financial. This advocacy may inappropriately extend to their medicolegal needs. Thus, some physicians who are called to testify believe wrongfully that it is their job to win the case for their patients.[4,5,7] In their zeal to do whatever they can to support their patient's legal claims, these doctors may minimize or even overlook relevant medical factors. Note the following:

Q.   Doctor, have you determined the cause of the patient's current pain symptoms?

A.   Yes.

Q.   And what is the cause?

A.   The cause of the patient's current condition is the traffic accident of last year.

Q.   Is last year's accident the sole cause of the patient's condition?

A.   Yes.

Q.   What about his previous back injury?

A.   What about it?

Q.   Don't you think the patient's previous back injury has some connection with this present pain problems?

A.   No, I don't think so.

Q.   Why not?

A. The previous back injury was five years ago. He had recovered from that injury and was working full-time as an air-conditioner repairman, but now he can't work at all. He's in a lot of debt because of last year's accident.

Q. Do you realize that, as a result of his back injury at work, he was rated 15% permanent partial disability with regard to his low back condition?

A. No. I didn't realize that.

Q. Given this information, don't you think that at least some current pain symptoms are caused by his previous work injury?

a. I'm not sure I can agree with that. I don't know how that disability rating was made. All I know is that he was working full-time until the car accident but since then he can't work at all. To me that means the car accident is the sole cause of his current pain problems.

The physician witness's adamant opinion that the car accident is the only cause of the patient's pain problems is untenable. The doctor's compassion for the patient's plight is misplaced, and the persistent denial of the pre-existing condition is wrong, borders on the unethical, presents the doctor as a hired gun, and will surely have an impact on the witness's credibility. The appropriate way to respond in this situation is to acknowledge the pre-existing injury, how the patient had recovered, albeit incompletely, and how the car accident affected the patient's condition.

Physicians who advocate for their patients in the courtroom can be readily identified by their tendency to overstate their opinions to reinforce the case, using extreme language such as:

a. There is no doubt in my mind . . .

a. I am absolutely certain . . .

a. In all the years I have been a doctor . . .

a. This is the worst case I've ever seen . . .

When expressed in such an exaggerated manner, the physician's testimony on behalf of the patient will be seen as biased and untrustworthy. More moderate positions expressed by the witness are found to have more credence, such as:

A. In my opinion . . .

A. The probability is . . .

A. The evidence leads me to conclude . . .

A. I believe . . .

As a medical witness, you want to remain objective, firmly express your opinions, defend your position, and advocate not for the patient but for the truth.[8]

Being Defensive

"Doctor, is there any excuse for the botched job you did?"
One of the ways a cross-examining attorney succeeds in reducing the witness's effectiveness is by stirring the expert's anxieties and defensiveness.[1,5] Note in the following exchange how the doctor's visceral reactions provide little help to the testimony.

Q. Doctor, when you saw the patient in the emergency room, you ordered a skull x-ray because of his head trauma, is that correct?

A. Yes.

Q. Did you order any blood tests?

A. No. I didn't.

Q. Did you order an electrocardiogram?

A. No. He didn't need an EKG. There was no concern about his heart.

Q. Did you order a CT scan of his head?

A. No. I didn't think it was necessary.

Q. Did you order an electroencephalogram?

A. No. I didn't think that was necessary, either.

Q. Did you order an MRI?

A. Of what?

Q. Of his head.

A. No.

Q. Doctor, we are talking about a man who sustained a significant head injury from a head-on car crash and who the next day fell into a coma and had to be hospitalized for two weeks. Why in the world didn't you do more for him than a simple x-ray?

a. Listen. You have no idea what you're asking. You just don't understand how emergency room physicians think and operate in the ER. When a person comes in after a car crash with a headache but is otherwise alert, oriented, and has no other complaints, the standard of practice in trauma medicine is to do what I did. It was a very busy night with bodies all over the place. I recall at least three people were on heart monitors because of chest pains, someone was bleeding from a knife wound in the abdomen, not to mention the other cuts and bruises we were attending to with a short staff. What I did was perfectly correct given the facts I had. Do you think it's right to order tests just because his car insurance will cover it? That's the kind of thinking that causes insurance rates to escalate and gives docs a bad name. Besides, in this era of managed care, if you dare to order an MRI for a headache the hospital will probably get stuck with the bill. Your question is thoughtless and shows your total ignorance about the realities of emergency room medicine.

This diatribe may trigger a sympathetic response in a juror or two, but for most the witness's angry outpouring far exceeded what was needed to answer the question and sounded more like excuses than an explanation. The witness box is not the place to grieve about emergency room pressures or proselytize about the health insurance crisis. A more prudent response would be

A. The actions I took when the patient appeared in the emergency room with headaches met with standard practices of medicine under those specific clinical conditions, which call for a thorough history and physical and head x-rays.

Being Disagreeable

"Doctor, do I detect a tone of negativism here?"
The cross-examination is designed to alter the expert witness's testimony in favor of the other side. For this purpose the opposing counsel will ask many questions, hoping to note some modifying or hedging of one's position, with questions such as:

Q. Doctor, don't you think the patient had a predisposition to have the medical condition that you attribute solely to the accident?

Q. Didn't his old injury from five years ago contribute to his present condition?

Q. If the patient followed her doctor's orders as initially prescribed, wouldn't she be in a better condition today?

The answer to questions like the above could be "No." However, it is unwise to be disagreeable and to simply answer "No" to any and all of the propositions offered by the opposing attorney. Your negativism will be apparent to the court and would cast doubt on your impartiality and judgment.

If an idea or question advanced by the cross-examiner has not been previously considered by the expert witness, then an appropriate response can be

A. I had not thought of that. Could I have some time to consider it?

The judge will doubtless give the expert a few minutes to think about the question, and the expert can return the following kinds of answers:

A. No. I don't think the old injury has anything to do with his present condition because . . .

A. Yes. It's possible that prompt attention to the doctor's orders would have helped, but overall I think the probability is low that she would be in a better condition today.

When the proposition offered by the cross-examiner is undeniably true, the response must be

A. Yes. That's true.

Accepting Authority of Books and Other Witnesses

"Isn't that the Bible truth?"

A cross-examiner may want the expert witness to endorse a well-known medical treatise or an eminent physician as being an *authoritative* source. The tactic here is to use any statement from the accepted authority to counter the medical witness's opinion so as to impeach the physician's testimony, as in this example:

Q. Doctor, do you recognize the book entitled *Harrison's Textbook of Medicine*?

A. Yes.

Q. Could you tell us about the book?

A. *Harrison's Textbook of Medicine* is one of the widely read textbooks in the field of internal medicine.

Q. I see. So, you would accept Harrison's text as an authoritative source, wouldn't you?

a. Yes. Of course.

A "Yes" answer gives blanket approval to the book and will obligate you to accept the opinions expressed in the text; if they conflict with any of your conclusions, your testimony may be jeopardized.[7-9] Do not accept any treatise as authoritative unless you are willing to accept the entire book as being accurate. Here are some alternatives to a "Yes" answer:

A. Although *Harrison's Textbook of Medicine* is a well-respected textbook in the field, there are other books that are also reliable authorities in this specialty.

A. I agree with much of what is written in *Harrison's Textbook of Medicine*, but not with everything.

A. I find *Harrison's* to be useful, but not in every single circumstance.

Be prepared to identify other books or the aspects of the book with which you disagree.

Another way to endanger your own testimony is to capitulate to the expertise of another medical witness whose credentials and years of experience may overshadow yours.[3,5] The opposing attorney will try to get a physician to defer to another expert, particularly when the physician is young or inexperienced in courtroom testifying. For example,

> Q. Doctor, you're familiar with the work of Dr. _____, aren't you?
>
> A. Yes. I am.
>
> Q. Could you tell the court who Dr. _____ is?
>
> A. He is Professor of _____ at the University of _____ Medical School. He is identified with his innovative work in the treatment of _____.
>
> Q. Has Dr. _____ published his research in _____?
>
> A. Yes. He has several articles and a well-known textbook.
>
> Q. Dr. _____ will be testifying in this trial. Wouldn't you defer to his expertise in this matter?
>
> a. Yes. Of course.

Even though other medical witnesses are superbly qualified based on their contributions to the field, you need not automatically defer to those witnesses any more than you would automatically defer to well-known textbooks. If you have formed a professional opinion based on firm grounds and reasoning, you are entitled to testify and present your own conclusions. You may, in fact, have more knowledge and valid opinions about the case than the so-called eminent scholar.

Changing Your Opinion

"What is the most current revision of your opinion?"
An experienced cross-examiner will coerce expert witnesses to alter or even retreat from their opinion by various means. Witnesses who change or abandon their opinions will be seen as unreliable and untrustworthy.[10] Note the following examples:

> Q. There are two medical experts who will testify in this case and offer conclusions very different from yours. Would this give you some pause as to your opinions in this matter?

a. I'm not sure. I would certainly respect the opinions of my medical colleagues.

Q. Would your opinion in any way change if you were told that the patient had abdominal pain for a month before his appendicitis was diagnosed?

a. If I knew that, I would probably have a different opinion.

Q. If you had the resources to conduct as many tests as there are available, don't you think you could have reached a different diagnosis?

a. More than likely, I would reach a different diagnosis.

Q. There has been testimony that your patient is a heavy drinker. Does that in any way change your opinion?

a. Yes. No doubt about it.

At first blush, the proper answer would appear to be to agree with the question. After all, a "No" response could suggest stubbornness, arrogance, or dogmatic thinking. However, a medical witness should not be too eager to acquiesce to the opposing lawyer's questioning. If you have reached valid findings based on solid evidence and cogent reasoning, you should stand firmly behind your testimony. Consider these preferred responses:

A. Although I respect the opinions of my colleagues, I would like to review their findings closely before I reconsider my position.

A. Not necessarily. It depends on what kind of abdominal pain he was reporting, where it was located, how long it lasted, and so forth.

A. It is ideal to be able to request every test in the book. But, in this case, the tests ordered were sufficient for me to make a firm diagnosis.

A. I need more information before I change my opinion. I need to know what he drinks, how much he drinks, how long he's been drinking, and if he has any of the sequelae of chronic alcoholism.

Of course, if new evidence comes to light that contradicts your conclusions, you should not hesitate to modify your position.

Letting Down Your Guard:

"One last thing, Doctor . . ."
Some attorneys will reserve an important question for the end of the cross-examination, when you may be relieved that the serious questioning is completed and you let down your guard. This is a version of a witness's mistake discussed earlier: not paying attention to each question.

Q. I thank you for your cooperation today, Doctor. I just have a few questions to wrap up, OK?

A. Sure.

Q. Medicine is a complex field, isn't it?

A. Yes, it is.

Q. That's why in this case you requested special consultants, like the cardiologist and the endocrinologist, right?

A. That's right.

Q. And you deferred to the cardiologist regarding the patient's heart condition, correct?

A. Yes.

Q. You have no opinion for us regarding the cause of the patient's heart condition, right?

A. Right.

Q. And no opinion regarding the cause of the patient's medical complications, right?

The exhausted and emotionally drained witness, eager to leave the witness stand and thinking that the essential questions have already been asked, might incorrectly answer, "Yes." If the "Yes" answer is in error, you might be rescued by your attorney who is aware of this courtroom tactic and will ask follow-up questions to salvage your testimony. Remember, do not let your guard down until you are dismissed as a witness.

Closing Arguments

While other chapters in this book familiarize you with the varied techniques and strategies of a cross-examining attorney, the present chapter focused on typical ways in which physician witnesses contribute to their own demise. These 10 ways to ruin your testimony should not be construed to be a "top 10" list or a complete list. Expert witnesses, being abundantly resourceful, can create as many original ways to self-destruct as there are expert witnesses. Although medical witnesses cannot control the kinds of formidable questions that an opposing lawyer may employ, they can at least avoid the self-injurious responses noted here.

References

1. Horsley JE. *Testifying in Court: A Guide for Physicians* (4th ed). Los Angeles: Product Management Information Corp., 1992.
2. Rossi FF. *Expert Witnesses*. Chicago: American Bar Association, 1991.
3. Appelbaum PS, Gutheil TG. *Clinical Handbook of Psychiatry and the Law* (2nd ed). Baltimore: Williams & Wilkins, 1991.
4. Liebenson HA. *You, the Expert Witness*. Mundelein, IL: Callaghan & Company, 1962.
5. Matson JV. *Effective Expert Witnessing: A Handbook for Technical Professionals*. Chelsea, MI: Lewis Publishers, 1990.
6. Moritz AR, Morris RC. *Handbook of Legal Medicine* (4th ed). St. Louis: CV Mosby, 1975.
7. Zobel HB, Rous SN. *Doctors and the Law*. New York: WW Norton, 1993.
8. Babitsky S, Mangraviti JJ Jr. *How to Excel during Cross-Examination: Techniques for Experts that Work*. Falmouth, MA: SEAK, 1997.
9. McGugin DE. Preparation for the Physician and Trial. In AE James (ed), *Legal Medicine: With Special Reference to Diagnostic Imaging*. Baltimore: Urban & Schwarzenberg, 1980.
10. Gee DJ, Mason JK. *The Courts and the Doctor*. Oxford, England: Oxford University Press, 1993.

6

Personal Injury:
Motor Vehicle Accidents and
Workers' Compensation

Personal injury lawsuits arise from tort claims that allege that a person, by negligence or by intention, inflicted injury on another person. A tort is simply an injury or damage to one's person, property, interests, or reputation.[1] Torts are private civil wrongs, in contrast to crimes, which are public wrongs. Whether a given tort claim evolves into a full-blown lawsuit depends on several factors, but paramount is the presence of real or perceived injury to the claimant, or plaintiff. The injury may be physical, emotional, or economic in nature or a combination of these, and when an injury occurs, the victim can seek monetary recompense from the person who allegedly caused it.

The claimant may be awarded special damages, which are compensation for financial losses, such as payment for medical care, hospitalization, and loss of wages. Sometimes the injured party is also awarded general damages for emotional injury, including anxiety, grief, and pain and suffering. On rare occasions the court awards punitive damages in the form of monetary fines or criminal punishment when the defendant's conduct has been grossly negligent or malicious.

If the defendant can prove that no injury was incurred by the plaintiff, then no award will be given. If the defendant can demonstrate that the actual injury suffered is less severe than claimed, then the amount of any damage awards would be determined accordingly. In general, the law deals more harshly when the injury is caused intentionally, such as in an assault, fraud, deceit, or defamation.[2]

Where an injury is truly accidental, that is, due to no one's fault, an injured person cannot ordinarily demand to be compensated.[3] It should be noted that this principle has been modified with certain insurance programs (e.g., workers' compensation), and the development of product liability laws that hold manufacturers and businesses liable for injuries resulting from use of products made or sold by them.[4] Under both strict workers' compensation insurance and liability approaches, compensation may be made in the absence of proof of fault or wrongdoing.[5]

In personal injury lawsuits, physicians play an essential role in determining the presence, the extent, the etiology, and the consequences of any physical injury.[6] Critics of the legal system often cite the disproportionate number of tort cases that involve medical injury or damage, with civil personal injury lawsuits often occupying 50–75% of the court calendar.[7] This phenomenon necessitates the frequent involvement of medical experts to resolve these disputed claims.

Tort claims can also involve physicians who fail in duties incident to their professional roles. Physicians are responsible for the safety and efficiency of the medicine, materials, and devices they employ. When a physician's conduct falls below the established standard of care expected of physicians and results in injury or damage, medical negligence can be claimed by the injured party. A physician commits an intentional tort when knowingly billing an insurance company for services not rendered. Finally, a physician, especially one who has a history of professional misconduct, may face punitive damages for any flagrant acts of medical negligence. See Chapter 7 for a full discussion of medical malpractice.

Motor Vehicle Accidents

A motor vehicle accident (MVA) is a prime example of a personal injury lawsuit. The major medicolegal issues usually consist of whether or not a defendant negligently caused a claimant's injuries and, if so, the extent and consequences of those injuries. Medical evidence is required to demonstrate the nature of the injuries, their causal relationship to the putative negligence, and their consequences to the claimant. The medical evidence typically includes medical records, diagnostic studies (e.g., x-ray studies, CT and MRI scans), reports, and oral testimony by physicians.

Considerable contention among attorneys and physicians arises over the well-known "whiplash" injury from an MVA.[8,9] Plaintiff attorneys contend that a whiplash injury may, despite few if any findings on physical and diagnostic studies, produce disabling neck pain associated with stiffness, headaches, dizziness, and personality changes. Defense-oriented attorneys, on the other hand, regard many claims of whiplash injuries as an attempt to convert an inconsequential injury into a large monetary award. Because of the complex nature of this kind of claim, it is often difficult to predict the fate of whiplash claims in litigation. Much will depend on the respective skills of the attorneys involved and the attitude of the insurers in settling these difficult claims.

In most communities, whiplash claims are big business in the field of personal injury law, and physicians will be caught in the crossfire between the opposing attorneys.[10,11] When a physician testifies for the claimant, the cross-examiner will seek to discount the claimant's symptoms and focus on the paucity of objective physical signs and diagnostic findings. Furthermore, the defense attorney often will suggest that the physician's interpretation of the claimant's symptoms is the result of the physician's failure to recognize the patient's secondary gain from the symptoms. A cross-examining lawyer's question in a whiplash case might proceed as follows:

Q. Doctor, you've testified that the patient has no definite physical findings and that her neck x-rays are negative. How then can you say that all these symptoms she complains of—neck pain, headache, and numb fingers—relate to the injuries that she allegedly incurred in the rear-end auto accident?

To answer this question the physician has to provide a careful exposition of concepts of how soft tissue injuries may produce muscle spasm and pain, how muscle spasm may alter superficial extracranial blood flow and produce headache, how functions of the upper cervical nerve roots can be disturbed and cause posterior or lateralized head pain, and how extensive soft tissue injuries, including ligament and muscle damage, may exist in the face of normal imaging studies (e.g., MRI scans). This type of answer provided by the physician is nonetheless vulnerable to contentions that the precise mechanisms by which many whiplash injuries produce symptoms are theoretical in nature, that the physician is offering only a speculation about pathophysiology, and that the claimant may simply be elaborating her symptoms for secondary gain, viz., financial profit. Even the physicians who are strongly convinced that a patient is suffering as a result of a whiplash injury often may not wish to endure this type of intensive legal inquiry.

A defense expert medical witness in a whiplash case may find it less stressful than being a plaintiff's expert because the typical whiplash case involves little in the way of objective or positive physical findings, and the physician can testify that the absence of abnormal signs on physical injury indicates that the plaintiff's symptoms have no organic or physical basis. Although the cross-examining plaintiff attorney may succeed in having the defense expert concede that not all real physical symptoms are accompanied by objective signs, the defense expert can assert that the lack of positive signs prevents one from concluding with reasonable medical probability that symptoms and injury are causally related. Medical testimony of this nature is difficult to shake on cross-examination.

When the physician's testimony is based on a rigid preconception that no whiplash injury ever produces persistent symptoms, an experienced plaintiff attorney will expose this bias and try to discredit the testimony in the eyes of the jury and judge. Additionally, some claimants can be effective in describing their symptoms in court; their vivid accounts of neck pain and tingling limbs may weigh more heavily with the jury and judge than the precise, but perhaps tedious, scientific testimony of the physician.

Following MVAs, similar diagnostic problems arise with respect to posttraumatic headache, posttraumatic neuralgia, causalgia, and low back pain. In these situations, clinical findings may be minimal or modest, great reliance is placed on the patient's subjective characterization of the pain experience, and the pathophysiologic mechanisms will be debatable. Furthermore, the medical witness must consider the intangible influences of individual perceptions and reactions to painful stimuli, as well as the psychological impact of involvement in a lawsuit and the role of secondary gain.

Medical testimony about chronic pain entails a careful and sensitive inquiry into the basis of a plaintiff's symptoms and the nature of the pain experience. With a thorough examination, the diligent and well-trained physician can reach a reasonable judgment about the nature of the symptom of pain. The court establishes the propriety of admitting into evidence the physician's opinions on these issues, and allows the judge and jury to determine whether or not the testimony is convincing.

When the physician states that a person is in pain, the cross-examiner will inevitably ask questions, such as:

Q. How do you know if a person is truly in pain?

Q. Can you measure the pain?

Various basic questions relating to pain must be answered in legal and administrative hearings:

"Does the claimant have pain?"

In view of the obvious financial interest in the outcome of a proceeding, the plaintiff's own statements about the pain experienced may not be credible to the jury and judge. Thus, the physician's testimony becomes crucial. Whenever a large monetary claim is involved, the physician who states that pain is present will have intensive cross-examination and face conflicting testimony by physicians testifying for the defense. Although pain is subjective and impossible to measure, the physician witness must be convinced about the presence or absence of pain and be convincing to the jury about the pain symptoms.

"Is the pain the result of the injury out of which the suit arose?"

This question goes to the heart of the issue of causation. Frequently, the defense counsel will try to establish that the plaintiff's symptoms were pre-existent, related to another disease/disorder, or a predisposition of the claimant's health condition. The plaintiff attorney can counter the issue of a pre-existing disease with the assertion that the injury aggravated or reactivated the condition. As for the presence of any predisposition, a legal precedent referred to as the "eggshell skull" principle has been helpful to plaintiff lawyers. This ruling states that a plaintiff who suffers more damage in an accident because of, say, a very thin skull cannot be held responsible simply because another person with a normally thick skull would have suffered less damage. In other words, a victim has to be taken as is.[12] The physician witness has the enormous task of concluding whether or not pain symptoms are causally linked to the injuries involved in the lawsuit.

"To what extent does the pain impair functional capacity or cause disability?"

Disability is a term employed in legal proceedings to quantify the impact of a given injury. The physician's role in this regard is to describe how a claimant's symptoms impinge on his or her vocational, social, and family activities. In the case of pain, the issues often are its limiting effect on various physical activities and its insidious implication of chronic suffering (i.e., how the pain affects the patient physically and psychologically). Individuals who conceive pain as a pre-eminently disagreeable experience agree that the emphasis of pain's psychological effects is a crucial issue.

"How long will the pain last?"

The physician will be asked to predict in these cases how long the pain will last. This opinion will be necessary to determine how much to award for future suffering. If the physician cannot, or will not, express his or her opinion in this regard, then no award can be made for this element of the legal case. The physician must also assess the extent to which pain relief can be achieved by medications or other techniques. If medical testimony indicates that pain will subside or can be effectively controlled by available treatments, then the amount of the monetary award for future suffering will be less.

"Could the patient be malingering?"

A medical examination of a plaintiff in a personal injury or workers' compensation lawsuit must consider the possibility of conscious or subconscious symptom magnification, secondary gain, compensation neurosis, and even faking, because the prospects of a substantial monetary windfall can influence the experience and presentation of symptoms such as pain. Unlike the clinician who noncritically accepts a patient's pain symptoms at face value, the medical expert must question the accuracy of the history and subjective complaints provided. In a forensic setting, the physician needs to obtain corroboration from unbiased external sources and should carefully investigate inconsistent symptom patterns and uncharacteristic complaints. However, in view of the fact that (1) medicine does not now have a precise measure of malingering, and (2) the accusation of faking has profound legal, financial, and other stigmatizing ramifications, the medical expert must be extremely cautious in making unqualified pronouncements regarding the veracity of individuals involved in litigation.

Workers' Compensation

Workers' compensation programs have been in existence since the turn of the century in response to the failure of the tort system to compensate workers adequately for injuries sustained in the course of their employment. These programs provide insurance to cover injury occurring at work, regardless of whether the injury is the result of the negligence or intentional fault of the employer.[13,14] Presently, the various states and the federal government have their own workers' compensation program with varying rules, coverage, and compensation schedules, with the amount of compensation varying according to the degree of injury.

In workers' compensation cases, a claimant's injury must be related to the job before an award can be considered. Thus, a worker who is injured while on a weekend or holiday will usually not be entitled to an award from the employer's insurer. Usually the concept of fault is not involved in a workers' compensation proceeding. The principle for allowing compensation is that employers have a duty to provide their employees a safe place to work and to arrange for insurance to cover those injuries occurring on the job. Hence, payment of compensation for work-related injuries will be mandated by state or federal statute, and the purpose of an administrative hearing will be to decide if a work-related injury occurred and how much compensation will be proper.

Often in workers' compensation cases the issue arises of an employee having an existing pathologic disease/condition that might have produced the disability, and at times death, regardless of the circumstances of employment.[15] Let us suppose a bank's vice president suffers an intracranial carotid aneurysm while sitting at his or her desk. The person would not receive compensation for any resulting disability because the cerebral aneurysm was a pre-existing condition, and there is no particular reason to believe that the circumstances of employment caused it to rupture. However, let us now suppose that the vice president's aneurysm ruptured while helping the office janitor move a heavy file cabinet. There have been cases allowing workers' compensation recovery for employees who sustain myocardial infarctions or strokes while engaged in activities beyond the usual demands of their employment. By analogy, a workers' compensation award might be made for the worker whose aneurysm ruptures while engaged in an unusual exertion, even though the clinical information about the role of exertion in causing aneurysms to rupture is inconclusive. Similarly, recovery of an award might be granted if the aneurysm ruptured while the employee was vomiting in response to inhalation of noxious fumes while on the job.

The physician who testifies in a workers' compensation case may be asked to opine whether or not an employee's pre-existing disorder was the sole or principal cause of an episode (e.g., subarachnoid hemorrhage) that occurred while at work. Where no specific stress or exertion existed at work, it would be difficult for the physician to relate the episode to employment. However, given proof of job stress or exertion, the physician can cite these as contributing factors. A more definitive statement might be sought early in the injured worker's treatment since the issue of the relationship of the injury to employment must be decided before disposition of an employee's claim can proceed. In this situation, without sufficient data the physician might feel forced to speculate; yet if the physician admits to be speculating, either directly or by not using terms such as "reasonable medical probability," the testimony may be discarded as insufficient to support a finding of causal connection between injury and employment.

Courtroom Examination

The courtroom examination of a physician in a personal injury lawsuit follows a format generally similar to that described in Chapters 3 and 4. As always, the first series of questions is aimed at establishing the physician's qualifications as an expert witness. After the physician has been qualified by the judge to testify as an expert, then the medical witness will be asked what background material pertaining to the patient was available for review, how the physical examination was conducted, what findings were obtained, and the causal link, if any, between the plaintiff's medical condition and the alleged incident.

The following examples of direct and cross-examination involve a hypothetical case of a man suffering injuries from a typical MVA. To facilitate reading, the examinations here contain the bare essentials and are much more concise than an actual courtroom testimony.

Direct Examination: Witness Qualification

In addition to the usual questions about the educational background and professional experience to qualify a physician as an expert witness, the physician witness can expect to answer the following pertinent questions:

Q. In your daily practice of medicine, do you have a special interest in (the specific kind of injury involved in the case)?

Q. Have you done any teaching or research in (the specific kind of injury involved in the case)?

Q. Have you ever testified in personal injury cases on behalf of
your patient?

Q. Have you ever testified in personal injury cases on behalf of
the defense?

Q. How often have you testified on behalf of your patients and
how often for the defense?

With regard to the last question, you may not know the exact numbers,
but it is helpful for the court to know in what capacities you have testified in previous personal injury cases. It is preferable, but not essential, that you have testified on both sides of a lawsuit, but it is critical
that you are impartial, objective, and professional in your role as an
expert witness.

The direct examination to qualify a witness is a typically straightforward formality of recording his or her medical credentials. For the
more experienced physician with significant accomplishments, this line
of inquiry will emphasize the impressive professional achievements that
qualify the physician as a recognized expert in the field. Thus, this initial questioning usually proceeds quickly and smoothly.

Cross-Examination: Voir Dire

After the physician's credentials have been verified on direct examination, the opposing lawyer has the opportunity to question the witness
in a voir dire procedure. The *voir dire* has a limited purpose of testing
and challenging the qualifications of the expert. The opposing counsel will try to flush out in cross-examination the limitations of your
competence by noting gaps in your professional training and work
experience. There may even be an attempt to disqualify you as a witness by claiming your lack of adequate credentials or by arguing that
your contribution is irrelevant or clearly biased. Accordingly, you can
anticipate the following kinds of questions aimed at discrediting you as
an expert:

Q. Your medical school background may sound impressive, but
you've had no special training in (the specific kind of injury
involved in the case), have you?

a. That's true. I can't argue that.

Q. Doctor, wouldn't you agree that your work as a clinician is more of an art than a science?

a. Of course, there's a lot of art in what doctors do.

Q. Doesn't your diagnosis involve a good deal of hunches and gut reactions?

a. We are never 100% sure in our diagnoses. Our hunches are based on years of experience and are important in our work with patients.

Q. Since you have testified in the past only for your patients, aren't you an advocate for them?

a. I'm an advocate for all my patients. I wouldn't be here if I didn't care about them.

The above answers are likely to diminish your credibility as a competent and objective witness. Instead of these impulsive and harmful statements, calmer and more thoughtful responses are clearly preferred, such as:

Q. Your medical school background may sound impressive, but you've had no special training in (the specific kind of injury involved in the case), have you?

A. My medical training has included several years of residency and continuing education covering the broad spectrum of health conditions. My training and experience give me the competence to treat (the specific kind of injury involved in the case) and many similar disorders.

Q. Doctor, wouldn't you agree that your work as a clinician is more of an art than a science?

A. I'm not sure what you mean by art, but my medical judgment is based on scientific principles as well as observable and quantifiable data. Medical practice is essentially scientific and not an art.

Q. Don't your diagnoses involve a good deal of hunches and gut reactions?

A. Hunches are helpful, but my diagnoses must be based on scientific facts and reasoning.

Q. Since you have testified in the past only for your patients, aren't you an advocate for them?

A. It's true that I've testified only for a patient in the past. However, if I were to be called by a defense lawyer to evaluate someone, I would have no objections to doing that.

Even when confronted with a vigorous *voir dire*, a physician witness is rarely disqualified from testifying. However, how well the doctor responds to this line of questioning may affect the weight given to the testimony.

Direct Examination of Plaintiff Witness

After being qualified by the judge to testify, the physician witness for the plaintiff will undergo the direct examination by the plaintiff attorney, who will elicit favorable testimony to support the contentions of the injured party. The plaintiff attorney and expert witness have probably conferred in advance of the trial and prepared questions that will enhance the conclusions of the physician witness.

Q. Doctor, have you ever treated a person by the name of Mr. Abel?

A. Yes, I have.

Q. When did you first see him?

A. On February 2 of this year.

Q. Who referred Mr. Abel to you?

A. He was referred by his family physician, Dr. Baker.

Q. Please tell us the history you obtained from Mr. Abel on February 2.

A. Mr. Abel told me that he was being referred to me because of his severe headaches as well as his neck and back pain. He had been treated by Dr. Baker who prescribed ibuprofen, a nonsteroidal anti-inflammatory drug, or NSAID, as well as physical therapy. He said he had these physical problems since last July when he was involved in a traffic accident in which the car he was driving was struck broadside on the passenger's side. Is this what you want?

Q. Yes. Please continue.

A. When his car was hit, Mr. Abel's head hit the door window. He lost consciousness briefly. He was taken by ambulance to a nearby hospital where he was examined, given some pain medications, and released with instructions to follow up with his regular doctor. A few days after the accident, because his headaches were quite painful, Mr. Abel saw Dr. Baker who prescribed the NSAID and cyclobenzaprine, and recommended physical therapy because of the neck and back pain he reported. He remained off work for a month, finding some relief of his neck pain with his physical therapy. He has been working full-time at the warehouse where he is a foreman though he is restricted to light duty, that is, not doing any heavy lifting over 50 pounds. Since the car accident he has had difficulty sleeping because of his headaches, and he reports being irritable and sensitive to loud noises.

Q. Can you tell us about your examination of Mr. Abel on February 2?

A. Yes. I did a complete physical examination and, except for a slight bump on the left side of his head and complaints of headaches, insomnia, and irritability, I found Mr. Abel to be normal.

Q. Did you conduct any test on Mr. Abel?

A. Yes. I requested a brain CT scan.

Q. What were the results of those tests?

A. Except for soft tissue swelling of the left parietotemporal scalp, the CT scan of Mr. Abel's brain was normal.

Q. What diagnoses did you reach on that first visit?

A. My diagnoses included a closed head injury with concussion and scalp contusion with residual posttraumatic headaches.

Q. What treatment have you provided for Mr. Abel's headaches?

A. I have prescribed an NSAID, naproxen, and amitriptyline.

Q. What has been his response to the treatment?

A. Mr. Abel's headaches improved as did his insomnia and irritability.

Q. What is your prognosis for Mr. Abel at this time?

A. I would say that the prognosis is fairly good. I expect continued infrequent headaches, less medication, and better moods.

Q. Doctor, do you have an opinion based on reasonable medical certainty as to what is causing Mr. Abel's headaches?

A. Yes.

Q. And what is that opinion?

A. The patient's headaches are the result of his injuries from the traffic accident of last July.

Q. Have you completed your treatment of Mr. Abel?

A. No. Although Mr. Abel has improved considerably since his first visit, I expect to see him for at least three more months because he still has painful headaches once a week, some upper back pain, and needs medications, such as naproxen and amitriptyline.

Q. After your treatment is completed, do you think he will need further medical assistance?

A. No.

Q. Thank you, Doctor. That's all the questions I have.

The physician witness has presented important medical information in an illuminating way. He explained the patient's injuries in everyday language that the average juror can understand, such as headaches, loss of sleep, and irritability. The clear testimony assists the jurors in understanding the medical issues of the case and they will appreciate the help of the expert witness.

Cross-Examination of Plaintiff Witness

The defense attorney has a duty to cross-examine the plaintiff witness in whatever manner to uncover weaknesses in the witness' statements, to discredit the witness's conclusions, and to reduce the impact of the witness's testimony. Areas of questioning may cover the following:

1. The bias of the treating physician

2. The pre-accident condition of the patient

3. The patient's pain experience

4. The base rates of symptoms

5. The patient's unreliable history

Physician Bias
"Are you testifying truthfully or just helping your patient?"

The treating physician who serves as an expert witness may be perceived as a biased advocate for his or her own patient. Thus, the following questions may emerge:

Q. Doctor, you are testifying here as Mr. Abel's treating physician, is that correct?

A. Yes.

Q. You have been his doctor for 9 months, right?

A. Yes.

Q. Now, the testimony you gave in the direct examination is helpful to your patient, isn't it?

a. Yes.

A "Yes" response is not desirable because it can be seen as an indication of a biased testimony in favor of the patient. A better response is

A. I don't know. Although I have been helping Mr. Abel with his medical problems, I am not here to help him with his legal claims.

or,

A. As a witness I am not testifying to help the patient but to help the jury with important medical information about the case.

Pre-Accident Condition
"Didn't he always have headaches?"

After the physician witness has linked the person's physical problems to a specific accident or incident, the defense attorney will often try to identify pre-accident health issues and nonaccident-related sources of symptoms. The following is a typical cross-examination approach:

Q. Doctor, you have been Mr. Abel's physician for the past 9 months, is that correct?

A. Yes.

Q. And in your opinion Mr. Abel's headaches, insomnia, and irritability were the result of the car accident of last July, is that right?

A. Yes.

Q. Doctor, did you have a chance to review the medical records of Dr. Charles, who was Mr. Abel's family doctor for many years?

A. No, I haven't.

Q. Did you know that Mr. Abel had previously complained of headaches and had been given muscle relaxants for several years?

A. No.

Q. Mr. Abel has been diagnosed as having high blood pressure, is that correct?

A. Yes.

Q. Don't people with high blood pressure often complain of headaches?

A. Yes, they do.

Q. If you know that Mr. Abel had problems with headaches long before last year's traffic accident, you would have some doubts as to whether the July car accident was the only cause of his current headache symptoms, wouldn't you?

a. I probably would.

Even though scheduled to testify in court, a treating physician is often not supplied with all of the patient's previous medical records.

Without complete pre-accident information, it may be presumptuous to connect specific physical symptoms to a single causal event. In this case, the physician witness could defend the conclusions by stating

    A. It may well be that Mr. Abel had headache problems in the past. Nonetheless, as far as I know, he was in good physical health and without headaches prior to the July accident, but he has had severe headaches ever since his head hit the car door window. This is why I believe his current condition is the direct result of the traffic accident last year.

Pain Experience
"Just how much pain does he really feel?"

To offset a plaintiff witness's testimony, the opposing attorney's strategy might be to emphasize the limitation of the witness's findings. The questioning method used by the lawyer is similar to the "chip away" strategy described by Rogers and Mitchell[16] in criminal forensic cases, as in the following:

    Q. Doctor, does Mr. Abel have headaches every day?

    A. No. He used to have daily headaches, but he now has headaches about once a week.

    Q. So, nearly every day he is headache-free, is that right?

    A. You could say that.

    Q. And when he does have that occasional headache, you've advised him to take some acetaminophen, right?

    A. That's right.

    Q. Acetaminophen reduces headache symptoms, correct?

    A. Yes.

    Q. In addition, Mr. Abel has been trained in relaxation techniques to control his headaches, isn't that true?

    A. Yes.

    Q. And he's been regularly using those techniques, right?

A. Yes.

Q. So, wouldn't you agree that when he has the occasional headache no more than once a week, they are markedly reduced by his headache medicine and relaxation methods?

A. Yes.

Q. Following your recommendations, how long do you think his headaches last?

A. Well, I'd say about a half hour to an hour.

Q. So, he is bothered by headaches about a half hour a week, is that right?

a. I haven't thought about his headaches in terms of time, but I guess your estimate is about right.

This relentlessly reductionistic approach by the opposing lawyer can be very effective. The above questions narrowly limited the subjective experience of pain while ignoring the widespread impact on the patient's life. The physician witness would do better by answering

A. I haven't thought about his headaches in terms of time. I think about his headaches in terms of how his life has been affected, how his headaches have caused him to avoid his usually active physical life, like working in the yard or playing with his children. He's missed work about 10 or 11 times, and he's never been known to have missed work before. He's gained more than 15 pounds probably because of his inactivity, and he feels like a totally different person.

Base Rates
"Don't we all have headaches?"

When interpreting groups of symptoms and arriving at diagnoses, health care providers have been known to overlook base rates, or the frequency with which symptoms occur in the general population. Ignoring base rates can lead a diagnostician to place greater significance on symptoms than is justified, a phenomenon referred to as "overpathologizing."[17] These false-positive diagnoses are misleading and will be challenged by the opposing attorney.

Q. Doctor, you have diagnosed Mr. Abel as having a postconcussion syndrome, is that right?

A. Yes.

Q. What do you mean by a postconcussion syndrome?

A. A postconcussion syndrome consists of a pattern of symptoms following head trauma, including headache, insomnia, fatigue, irritability, anxiety, and problems with concentration and memory.

Q. Are headaches an important feature of a postconcussion syndrome?

A. Yes.

Q. Did you know that in a survey of 1,200 adults, 70% of the respondents experienced headaches?

A. No. I'm not familiar with that survey.

Q. Isn't it true that many people without head injury have sleep problems of one kind or another?

A. That's true.

Q. And isn't irritability commonly experienced by many every day?

A. Yes.

Q. Doctor, wouldn't you agree that the symptoms Mr. Abel is reporting, such as headaches, sleep problems, and irritability, are the same as those who haven't had any head injury?

a. I can't argue with that.

When a patient has health problems that are no different than any normal individual, the patient has no claim to damages for an accident. In the above example, Mr. Abel may well be exhibiting a postconcussion syndrome, and the physician witness would do better by replying

A. It is true that headaches, sleep problems, and irritability are experienced by many people without head injury, but this person did not have any of these symptoms before the July accident and reported having these problems immediately after his head injury. Moreover he had neck and back pain and increased sensitivity to loud noises. I do not think that this combination of symptoms occurs often in the average person.

Unreliable History
"How accurate can a plaintiff's story be?"

All physicians rely to some extent on the history provided by the patient. Because there are factors that can distort a person's recollection of the past, including a fallible memory or even financial interests in a lawsuit, opposing lawyers frequently focus on the amount of weight given to potentially inaccurate medical history.

Q. Isn't it true that some medical cases are clear-cut in terms of making a diagnosis because of the abundance of objective test findings, such as CT scans?

A. That's true.

Q. In this case, can you tell us what percentage of your opinion was based on the historical data pertaining to the patient and what percentage was based on medical tests?

A. That's difficult to say. I'd guess about fifty-fifty.

Q. As far as historical information is concerned, you have relied on the facts as given to you by Mr. Abel, isn't that true?

A. That's true.

Q. So, Doctor, if what is told to you is inaccurate, you couldn't reach a conclusion, right?

a. Yes. That's right.

The attorney may discontinue this line of questioning, having accomplished the goal of demonstrating that the information the physician relied on was provided by a self-serving plaintiff. It is better to respond by denying that your conclusions were based primarily on what the plaintiff has said.

A. My conclusions are based on several factors, including what the patient told me, but also a review of his medical records, my clinical examination of him, and the various diagnostic tests I ordered. (Be prepared to provide specific details from the medical records and your examination of the patient.)

Direct Examination of Defense Witness

The physician who is a witness for the defense will undergo questioning by the attorneys on both sides regarding his or her competence to offer expert testimony. The defense attorney will, of course, ask questions that will highlight the physician's professional credentials. On the other side, the plaintiff attorney will try to emphasize the relatively brief contact the defense doctor has had with the patient compared with the treating physician who has seen the patient many times over a longer period of time. The plaintiff attorney might suggest possible witness bias if the physician has worked for the defense attorney in the past or bring out locality issues if the defense witness is from out of town and perhaps unfamiliar with the health practices and idiosyncracies of the hometown community. The voir dire challenges may affect how well the jury accepts the defense witness, but with rare exception the physician will be permitted to testify before the court.

Like the opposing side has done, the defense attorney and defense witness have probably met before the trial to prepare questions that will best present the arguments for the defense. A typical direct examination of a defense witness would include the following:

Q. Doctor, at my request did you see and do an independent medical examination of Mr. Abel?

A. Yes, I did.

Q. Can you tell us what the examination consisted of?

A. First, I received all of the medical records your office sent me before my appointment with Mr. Abel. My examination of him involved a 1-hour interview and a comprehensive physical examination. I also ordered a CT scan of his head, neck, and back.

Q. Doctor, based on all of the medical records you have reviewed as well as your interview and examination of Mr. Abel, did you reach an opinion based on a reasonable degree of medical certainty as to what his condition is?

A. Yes.

Q. Please tell the court and jury what your conclusions are.

A. In my opinion, Mr. Abel exhibits no significant health problem at this time. In other words, my evaluation of him produced normal results.

Q. Doctor, of what significance is the patient's reporting of headaches?

A. The patient has very mild headaches that occur no more than once a week and are readily reduced by taking nonprescription acetaminophen.

Q. What about his sleep problems?

A. He says he sleeps 5 hours a night. He does not seem to be affected much by this as he has been working full-time for the past year or more.

Q. What do you make of his irritability?

A. All of his symptoms—headache, insomnia, and irritability— are very subjective. They do not appear to be significant. Certainly he doesn't need a psychiatrist for his irritability.

Cross-Examination of Defense Witness

After the defense witness's direct examination is completed, the plaintiff's attorney has the task of challenging the defense witness's statements and attacking the troublesome areas of testimony. The cross-examination may include the following issues:

1. The limited information obtained by the expert witness

2. The incomplete testing done by the expert witness

3. Hypothetical questioning

4. The "hired gun" stigma

5. Witness's fees

Limited Information
"You hardly know the patient, right?"
The plaintiff attorney will try to show that the defense witness has had limited contact with the case and may not be as familiar with the patient as the treating physician. The following cross-examination may occur:

Q. Doctor, in performing your evaluation of this case, did you talk to Dr. Charles, the patient's family doctor?

A. No, I did not.

Q. Did you speak with Mrs. Abel, the patient's wife, or Mr. Abel's employer?

A. No, I didn't.

Q. How many times did you actually see Mr. Abel?

A. I saw him one time.

Q. And how long was your examination of him?

A. About an hour and a half.

Q. Wouldn't you agree that a doctor who has treated the patient many times over a 9-month period, who has spoken with his family physician, his wife, and his employer, has much more information about the patient than you do?

a. Yes. I would agree.

The "Yes" answer supports the plaintiff attorney's viewpoint that the defense expert has less information than the treating physician and thus may have less valid opinions about the case. If the defense witness has done a thorough evaluation, the following reply is appropriate:

A. I have had an abundance of data available to me including all of Mr. Abel's previous medical records, with the many tests performed since his accident. With that and the physical examination I performed, I had more than sufficient information on which to base my opinions with confidence.

Incomplete Testing
"You didn't even do a blood test?"

Because of practical considerations (e.g., time and finances), the physician witness may not have conducted the most ideal and comprehensive examination. Thus, questions may be designed to imply that the evaluation was incomplete and inadequate.

Q. You testified that the patient was not medically impaired, is that correct?

A. Yes.

Q. You based your conclusions on the records review and your examination of him, right?

A. Yes.

Q. You ordered a CT scan of his head, right?

A. Yes.

Q. Did you order an EEG?

A. No, I didn't.

Q. Did you request an MRI scan of his head?

A. No, I didn't.

Q. Did you request any neuropsychological testing?

A. No.

Q. Isn't it true that the results from an EEG, MRI, and neuropsychological testing could have been very helpful in reaching your conclusions?

a. That's true.

Q. I realize that you had to travel from out of town. If you had more time with the patient you could have obtained more information that would help you know the patient better, isn't that true?

a. Yes. That's true.

Agreement to the last two questions raises the possibility that the physician's conclusions were derived without a complete examination. If the witness has done a sufficiently thorough examination, a better reply would be

A. Additional information is always helpful, but I believe I performed a complete examination and did not need more information to reach my conclusions.

Hypothetical Question
"Assume the patient was never in an accident . . ."

Attorneys often employ hypothetical questions to elicit statements favorable to their side of the argument. The opposing counsel may object to the hypothetical question (e.g., if it assumes inaccurate facts), but the witness may be requested to answer the questions as posed by the attorney.

> **Q.** Doctor, I want to ask a question based on the following: Assume that Mr. Abel was in a traffic accident, striking the left side of his head and suddenly developing severe headaches that are improved but persist to the present time. Further assume that when he does occasional yard work or repair work at home, his headaches become more frequent and severe. Finally, assume that Mr. Abel never missed work for four years before the car accident, but since the injuries he sustained in the traffic collision, he has missed work eleven days in the past year because of painful, debilitating headaches. Given these assumptions, is it likely or unlikely that Mr. Abel has suffered posttraumatic headaches as a result of the car accident last year?

> **a.** It's likely he has suffered posttraumatic headaches from the car accident.

The hypothetical question is usually composed of true facts that the questioning attorney can support. However, to simply agree with the hypothetical question can contradict your previous testimony. Because you are not absolutely sure about the accuracy of the assumptions in the hypothetical question, you are advised to offer an appropriate disclaimer in your response.

> **A.** Assuming what you have said is true, it would appear likely that Mr. Abel suffered posttraumatic headaches from the car accident.

You may also state that you cannot answer the question because there is insufficient information to formulate an opinion, but you may then be asked to indicate what other information is needed for the hypothetical question to be answerable.

Hired Gun
"If you're hired, then you're a hired gun, correct?"
The expert witness who is retained by a law firm specifically to testify in court may have the appearance of being a "hired gun," who is paid handsome fees to present testimony favorable to one side. The plaintiff

attorney will pursue this line of inquiry aggressively, especially if the witness has been retained by the same lawyer in the past.

Q. Doctor, have you been hired by the defense attorney in the past?

A. Yes, I have.

Q. How many times have you worked for his law firm?

A. About four or five times.

Q. Have you been hired by other defense attorneys?

A. Yes.

Q. And how many times have you testified for other defense attorneys?

A. About 10 times.

Q. Have you ever testified for a plaintiff?

A. Yes. About five or six times.

Q. Isn't it true that your opinions are favored by defense attorneys who hire you more often?

a. It seems that way.

This response seems to agree with the implications that the witness's testimony is slanted toward the defense. When the physician's evaluation and opinions are grounded in solid medical evidence, then the reply should be

A. I don't know who favors my opinions. I know that I base my conclusions on objective medical evidence and it is my duty to be an impartial medical expert who favors neither side of a case.

Witness's Fees
"Aren't you being paid more than the judge?"

Questions about fees being paid for expert witnesses frequently emerge as a way to portray the witness as a mercenary rather than a highly competent professional.

Q. Are you being paid for the time you spend on this case?

A. Yes, I am.

Q. What is your fee?

A. It's $250 per hour.

Q. How do you determine your fee?

A. My fee represents the amount I would be earning if I were seeing patients in my office.

Q. Aren't your opinions influenced by the fact that you are being paid by the defense?

A. Absolutely not.

Q. Is your fee the same for testifying in court today?

A. No. My fee for courtroom appearances is $350 per hour.

Q. Why is there a difference between your consultation fee and your testifying fee?

a. Most doctors do that. I think it's because we don't like to testify in court.

This response may be true but quite inadequate. The jury would prefer a better explanation about one's legal fees.

A. Several reasons. Testifying in court is a much more demanding and rigorous process. The unpredictable scheduling of my appearance in court usually results in some lost time. Thus, I feel compelled to charge more to come to court than to review records or talk with attorneys on the phone.

Closing Arguments

The current trend in our litigious society to sue for any undesirable occurrence has sharply increased the need for health care professionals to testify in court. In addition to everyday slips and falls and fender benders, other catastrophes such as airline mishaps, bomb explosions, and building fires immediately result in hundreds of victims who are physically injured and who seek not only medical treatment but also financial compensation for their putative medical damages.

This chapter, focusing on personal injury or tort litigation, emphasized the controversies that arise out of mild whiplash injuries when the patient reports long-lasting neck pain and other medical symptoms in the absence of solid physical and diagnostic findings. Workers' compensation cases present similar medicolegal issues, with the physician having to prove that the circumstances of employment produced the employee's medical disability. In view of these perplexing issues, the physician witness needs to conduct an evaluation that is more comprehensive than the ordinary office visit. The physician must be knowledgeable about the claimant's preinjury medical status and any nonaccident health factors.

Treating physicians who become witnesses for plaintiffs face vigorous cross-examination that raises questions about the treating physician's bias, the patient's pre-accident condition, the patient's pain experience, the base rates of symptoms, and the patient's unreliable history. The physicians retained by the defense encounter other penetrating questions about the limited information obtained by the expert witness, the incomplete testing done by the expert witness, hypothetical questions, the "hired gun" stigma, and witness's fees.

Physicians who treat persons involved in tort litigation have important responsibilities when their patients' lawsuits require their professional documentation and explanation. In these personal injury cases, the physician being called as an expert medical witness will need to ask, "Am I really an expert on the issues in question?" For example, a general surgeon might be an ideal expert witness in a case of injury involving surgical intervention but not if the primary claim is of psychiatric impairment. If any doubt exists, the prudent decision is to decline testifying as an expert.

When the civil lawsuit involves substantial damages and high monetary stakes, physician witnesses can expect intense cross-examinations from highly paid and skillful attorneys. No wonder then that, if at all possible, physicians avoid involvement in legal testimony. However, for the well-prepared professional, courtroom testifying is a valuable contribution to the jurisprudence process and can be a challenging and rewarding experience for the physician.

References

1. Wade JW, Schwartz VE, Kelly K, Partlett DF (eds). *Prosser, Wade and Schwartz's Cases and Materials on Torts*. Westbury, NY: The Foundation Press, 1994.

2. Hoffman AC. Torts. In American College of Legal Medicine (ed), *Legal Medicine: Legal Dynamics of Medical Encounters*. St. Louis: CV Mosby, 1988;34–46.
3. Loimer H, Guarnieri M. Accidents and acts of God: a history of terms. *Am J Public Health* 1996;86:101–107.
4. Robertson LS. *Injury Epidemiology*. New York: Oxford University Press, 1992.
5. Ginnow AW, Nikolic M. *Corpus Juris Secundum* (Vol 1A). St. Paul, MN: West Publishing, 1985.
6. Karhu LA. Performing a workers' compensation medicolegal evaluation. *J Am Podiatr Med Assoc* 1995;5:149–153.
7. Beresford HR. *Legal Aspects of Neurologic Practice. Contemporary Neurology Series*. Philadelphia: FA Davis, 1975.
8. Sturzenegger M, DiStefano G, Radanov BP, Schnidrig A. Presenting symptoms and signs after whiplash injury: the influence of accident mechanisms. *Neurology* 1994;44:688–693.
9. Frankel CJ, Averbach A, McNeal HJ. "Whiplash" injuries. *Tenn Law Rev* 1961;29:157.
10. Wecht CH. Use and abuse of medicolegal and forensic scientific expert testimony in the courtroom. *Med Law* 1996;15:43–63.
11. Gotten N. Survey of 100 cases of whiplash injury after settlement of litigation. *JAMA* 1956;162:865.
12. Harrison GL. Psychiatry. In JP Jackson (ed), *A Practical Guide to Medicine and the Law*. London: Springer-Verlag, 1991;217–238.
13. Schmulowitz J. Workers' compensation: coverage, benefits and costs, 1992–93. *Social Security Bull* 1995;58:51–57.
14. Ringen K, Pollack E, Finklea JF, et al. Health insurance and workers' compensation: the delivery of medical and rehabilitation services for construction workers. *Occup Med* 1995;10:108–111.
15. Long AB, Brown RS Jr. Workers' compensation introduction for physicians. *Va Med Q* 1995;122(2):108–111.
16. Rogers R, Mitchell CN. *Mental Health Experts and the Criminal Courts*. Scarborough, Ontario: Carswell Thomson Professional Publishing Canada, 1991.
17. Faust D, Ziskin J, Hiers JB. *Brain Damage Claims: Coping with Neuropsychological Evidence*. Los Angeles: Law and Psychology Press, 1991.

7

Medical Malpractice:
The Expert Witness
and the Physician-Defendant

The first recorded lawsuit for medical negligence in America occurred in Connecticut in 1794. Over the past 200 years there have been countless instances in which patients sued their doctors to recover damages for injuries alleged to be the result of medical malpractice. In recent decades an astonishing increase has occurred in the number of medical malpractice lawsuits brought against physicians and health care facilities. A variety of forces in our society have transformed the traditional doctor-patient relationship: Consumerism, cynicism, mistrust of physicians' motivations, and the inevitability of less-than-perfect treatment outcomes have combined to make it relatively easy for individuals to consider suing their doctors. Highly sophisticated and complex medical technology with its attendant increased risks and greater expectations for perfect results can also claim partial responsibility for this phenomenon.[1] Moreover, medical malpractice litigation is a potentially lucrative endeavor for plaintiffs and attorneys as evidenced by escalating jury awards and associated legal contingency fees.[2]

Several questions occur to the physician when the issue of medical malpractice is raised:

- What constitutes a medical malpractice claim?

- When is a physician negligent in the duty to care?

- How is medical negligence proved?

- Who can be an expert witness in a medical malpractice lawsuit?

What Constitutes a Medical Malpractice Claim?

A medical malpractice lawsuit is one that claims negligence on the part of the physician in the performance of a medical act. In a medical negligence suit, the plaintiff must prove certain basic facts[3-5]:

1.   The physician had a duty to care for the plaintiff. The essential point to be established is the intention of the physician to advise, diagnose, or treat the plaintiff, with the duty persisting until the need for care no longer exists or until alternative arrangements have been made.

2.   The physician failed in the duty to care. Failure is determined when the medical services provided fall below generally accepted standards of practice.

3.   The failure to provide appropriate care was a proximate cause of the injury to the plaintiff.

4.   The injury or loss can be measured for compensation in money damages. The court will be interested in the severity of the injury, the prognosis, and the practical implications of the injury.

When Is a Physician Negligent in the Duty to Care?

For a claim of medical negligence to be proven, the plaintiff's attorney must be able to demonstrate one of several possibilities:

1.   The physician departed from commonly accepted standards of medical practice. Not all deviations from common professional practice are evidence of negligence. A slight, and at times significant, departure from the standard medical textbook treatment is not necessarily negligence, given the unique circumstances of each individual patient as well as the rapid pace of changing technologies and the delays in medical publications. Although the medical defendant may not follow the majority standard, that is, how most physicians perform the action being analyzed, the physician must at least follow the standard of what is called the respected minority. Every new treatment technique is a departure from accepted practice but does not necessarily constitute an act of negligence. Accepted practice may differ from one community to another and from one situation to another (e.g., intensive care unit ver-

sus accident scene). The important question is whether the method of diagnosis and treatment was or was not reasonable. The physician who provides inadequate reasons for departing from the normal procedures is one who is vulnerable to charges of negligence.

2. The physician failed to keep abreast with changes in medical practice. This may appear self-evident but it is not easy to prove exactly when an old method becomes obsolete and inadequate.

3. The physician employed a new but unproved and unaccepted method of treatment. If a novel method is used, the physician must be able to show that the traditional treatment is inferior to the new technique and that the anticipated risks of the new method are overshadowed by the potential benefits. The courts will reject procedures that are ostensibly radical or bizarre.

4. The physician did not take precautions against risks. For example, the use of Pantopaque in myelography was not a foreseeable risk in 1960, but it is now no longer used because of the foreseeable risk and negligence recognized in the 1990s.

5. The physician did not perform to the standards expected of his or her specialty. A general practitioner must be judged by the standards of other general practitioners, not of specialists. However, if the general practitioner attempted a specialist's task, the general practitioner would be judged by the standards of that specialty. Within a specialty field, the standard of care is that of the *reasonably competent specialist,* not that of the most experienced or the least qualified specialist.

When considering medical negligence, plaintiffs and the courts must be reminded that no cure is guaranteed in medicine, that a medical complication is not synonymous with medical negligence, that there is often more than one accepted method of treatment, and that physicians are not held to the highest standard in their specialty but are required to meet the standard of ordinary care or the accepted practice in the community.[6] Thus, a physician who performs in accordance with the commonly accepted practice of other physicians in similar circumstances will not be held to have been negligent. In addition, the physician is not liable for an incorrect diagnosis, provided the physician has obtained a careful history, made a thorough examination of the patient, used appropriate diagnostic tests, and exercised reasonable medical judgment. Finally, the court will make appropriate allowances when a physician has acted under emergency circumstances.

On occasion the court may determine that a commonly accepted practice is negligent. For example, a physician could be following a practice for reasons such as habit, convenience, or cost while seemingly subordinating risk factors for the patient. However, for a generally accepted standard to be condemned as negligence is extremely rare.

How Is Medical Negligence Proved?

The burden of proving that a physician was negligent rests with the plaintiff and the plaintiff's attorney. Physician-defendants are not obligated to prove that they were not negligent. The standard of proof required in medical negligence cases is the normal standard for civil tort: "preponderance of the evidence" or "more likely than not." The standard differs from the higher standard required for criminal justice cases, which is "beyond a reasonable doubt."

The plaintiff's attorney must prove a causal link between the physician's breach of duty and the damage sustained by the plaintiff. To prove causation, attorneys often rely on an approach known as the "but for" test. If the damage to the plaintiff would not have occurred "but for" the physician's negligence, then the negligence is considered a cause of the damage. For instance, in an elective cholecystectomy, if the surgeon injures the bile duct or liver by faulty surgical treatment, this negligence would be the cause of the damage to the patient. The plaintiff's attorney would argue that "but for" the surgical negligence the patient would be healthy.

The testimony of a medical expert witness is a vital ingredient necessary for a medical malpractice case to be successfully executed. A medical expert witness becomes necessary to establish in the minds of the judge and jury that the physician-defendant violated standards of care. An attorney who is presented with a potential medical malpractice claim needs to determine the merits of the case and sometimes will consult a physician or a certified registered nurse for this purpose. Thus, even before a case is accepted or a legal claim filed, a physician may be retained to assess whether the case has a reasonable chance of success.

Once a malpractice claim is filed, attorneys engage in a discovery process, or pretrial investigatory procedures, to obtain essential supporting documents and witness statements. As part of the discovery process, attorneys on both the plaintiff and defense sides can question witnesses to be called on in the case. A physician witness will probably be questioned by undergoing an oral deposition, which is a sworn testimony obtained in the presence of attorneys from both sides and recorded by a court reporter. (A more complete explanation of depositions and guidelines for the physician giving a deposition are presented in Chapter 9.)

The testimony of the medical expert witness is essential. Without it the plaintiff has no case. In a medical malpractice case, the physician witness will define the relevant standards of medical care, testify whether the physician-defendant deviated from that standard, and provide evidence and arguments that establish a causal link between the breach of duty and the plaintiff's medical damages. Opposing lawyers will challenge these conclusions and most probably retain their own medical expert to offset the testimony of the other side. Our legal adversary system of debating opposite opinions determines how the malpractice case will ultimately be resolved.

There are certain situations in which medical expert testimony is not required to establish proof of negligence. These are instances of medical negligence when the carelessness of the physician would be obvious to any layperson. Examples would be when a surgical sponge is left in the patient's body, when the wrong extremity is amputated, or when basic diagnostic tests, such as x-ray films for a bone fracture, are not used. In these cases, the doctrine of *res ipsa loquitur* (the thing speaks for itself) applies, acknowledging that the accident clearly could not have happened unless someone was negligent.[7] Although a medical expert witness may not be needed, physician-defendants have the right to challenge the presumptions of negligence with their explanations or with expert witnesses.

Who Can Be an Expert Witness in a Medical Malpractice Suit?

Several factors must be considered when an attorney selects a physician to serve as an expert witness in a medical malpractice lawsuit. The most important characteristics of an effective medical witness are the expert's qualifications (i.e., educational background, overall knowledge, and experience in the specific field of medicine). It is important that the medical witness devotes a considerable percentage of professional time to the specialty that is the focus of the litigation.

In most jurisdictions, the physician witness need not be practicing the medical specialty at issue to qualify as an expert witness. For example, a general internist who is familiar with but is not a specialist in cardiology could conceivably qualify to offer expert testimony in a cardiology case. However, the lack of board certification in cardiology may affect the weight given to the internist's testimony.

Statutes regarding medical expert witnesses differ among the varied jurisdictions. In some states, for example, the physician witness must have knowledge of the same school of practice ("the same school rule") and even have familiarity with the medical standards in the same or similar geographic region ("the locality rule"). Other states require that the physician witness be familiar with the standards of care pertaining to the time period of the case in litigation ("the contemporaneous practice rule"). Texas, for example, has established evidentiary rules requiring that physician experts prove familiarity with the standards of practice during the relevant time frame.[8]

Some states even require a physician witness to have a certain number of years of practice and medical experience in a particular medical specialty, with proven knowledge of the standards of care applicable to the specialty ("the same specialty rule"). In California, for example, physicians with experience in emergency medicine are the only experts qualified to appear against an emergency physician in a medical malpractice lawsuit.[4]

Expert Witness versus Professional Witness

In searching for an ideal medical expert witness in a medical malpractice case, lawyers sometimes prefer a local physician who may seem more credible to the jurors than an authority from out of town. However, plaintiff attorneys often have difficulty finding local physicians who are willing to testify against their colleagues. Physicians find it extremely distasteful to testify against fellow physicians, against those who have been sources of referrals, or against hospitals where they have staff privileges. Consequently, in many instances the plaintiff's counsel has no choice but to hire a physician expert from outside the community.

The out-of-town physician has the advantage of being unhindered by conflicts of interest, except for the perceived bias for being retained by one side. The outsider can be more objective and less affected by the pressure not to harm or betray known colleagues and associated hospitals. Some outsiders also benefit from a halo effect as an authority figure from a big city or university medical center. The average lay juror, however, may at times be unreceptive to a physician who does not share the same regional viewpoints and accents as the home folks.

A physician who is a member of the faculty of a major teaching institution has immediate appeal to most jurors. Furthermore, an expert who has published scientific articles, chapters, or books will also be highly regarded in court. Clinicians who are not involved in research or teaching can still be valid witnesses, but their perceived value would pale in comparison to that of an opposing academic scholar.

At times the choice will be between a physician who specializes in legal medicine and a full-time medical practitioner. *Professional witnesses* who devote more time to medicolegal cases than to medical practice have the forensic advantage as a result of their experience and skills in the courtroom. They have the ability to grasp the core medical issues, to present their opinions in a cohesive and convincing manner, and to cope with the various tactics of the trial attorney. Professional witnesses appear in any civil tort case, such as those involving motor vehicle accidents, but may be even more valued by some lawyers in medical malpractice lawsuits in which the scientific issues are complex and the stakes high.

There are certain disadvantages in employing a physician who specializes in legal medicine. For example, an experienced professional witness could be confronted with transcripts or videotapes from previous trials or depositions which contain responses that are inconsistent with the present testimony. Much can be made by a veteran trial counsel of even a minor inconsistency, which can offset an otherwise credible courtroom testimony. Questioning of professional witnesses may reveal that they earn a lucrative annual income from their forensic activity and that they obtain most of their revenue from one side of court cases, working solely for plaintiffs' attorneys or for the defense.[9] Such forensic specialists may be perceived as merely a hired gun or mouthpiece for the attorney. Furthermore, because of their part-time practice of medicine, professional witnesses may be considered less than an expert in difficult or controversial medical matters. Some professional witnesses have the reputation of being popular among attorneys because of their cooperative spirit and tendency to shape their testimony according to the needs of the attorney that employs them. They may be willing to provide favorable testimony for the right fee, even when it entails a departure from scientific methodology.[10] These witnesses clearly deserve the pejorative label of "hired gun."

The reluctance of physicians to testify against medical colleagues except in the most flagrant of circumstances has often made it necessary for lawyers to solicit assistance in their case presentation from medical practitioners who fall short of the best standards of the properly qualified medical witness. It is not unusual for physician witnesses to give testimony germane to a specialty other than the one in which they practice. Professional medical witnesses sometimes purchase advertising space in legal publications and bar journals stating "Doctor available to testify in medical malpractice cases."[11] Such advertisements may result in more medicolegal referrals, but they also supply the opposing attorney with an opportunity to depict the physician witness as one whose opinions can be bought.

Ideally, the medical expert witness is one who renders an unbiased professional opinion that is based on thorough training, personal experience, a firm knowledge of current medical practices, and an in-depth familiarity with the facts of the case at hand. He or she will testify based on an appreciation of civic duty rather than on the basis of economic remuneration to be determined by the outcome of the case that is decided on the weight of that expert's testimony. Physicians who are considering becoming medical experts must also determine if they can devote sufficient time and energy to these complex medicolegal actions.

Frequently, a qualified physician will wonder whether it is right to testify as an expert witness in a malpractice proceeding. Others may question if it is appropriate to refuse to testify in any medical malpractice case. The jurisprudence system has been designed to seek out what is true and what is fair. Physicians, like all citizens, have a civic obligation to aid justice, and the obligation is even greater when the physician's testimony becomes essential to a case, such as when the physician is the only specialist in the community. This ethical duty to testify under these circumstances applies not only to medical malpractice cases but in any legal action.[7] There can be no valid charge of impropriety leveled at medical witnesses when physicians offer their expertise to assist the courts in the discovery of truth. It is when the expert witness's inducements move toward mercenary or malevolent quests that valid objections can and should be raised.

It becomes a personal decision whether to ever participate as an expert medical witness. The physician must ensure that fear, apathy, or cynicism is not the driving force behind the choice not to be involved. Our current legal system cannot function well without the input of qualified physicians. Physicians who are willing to testify not only on behalf of good medical practices, but also in opposition to bad medical practices demonstrate to the medical profession and to a skeptical public that physicians are not involved in a "conspiracy of silence," but are dedicated to the fundamental principle of protecting the safety of patients.

Expert Witness in a Medical Malpractice Case

Trial Preparation

The physician who agrees to serve as an expert witness in a medical malpractice case will receive from the attorney voluminous clinical records as well as deposition transcripts obtained earlier from the physician-defendant, plaintiff, and witnesses. This is accompanied by a cover letter, sometimes summarizing the case. The physician's responsibility is to carefully read the documents; tab relevant pages; and take notes of critical events, progress notes, medication usage, test results, and any hospitalizations and surgical procedures. Sometimes more information is needed, such as job evaluations or school transcripts, and these should be requested from the attorney.

A close working relationship with the referring attorney is essential. After the medical documents have been reviewed, the attorney may want to discuss the case on the telephone or in person, avoiding a written opinion that can be discovered by the other side. If the physician's preliminary opinions are of no value or are harmful to the client's case, the attorney has the right not to employ the physician as an expert witness. If the medical opinion appears helpful to the case, a written opinion will be requested. When there are plans for the physician to do further investigation, such as a clinical evaluation of the patient, a written report will be submitted after all examinations and tests are completed.

The next phase for the medical witness will probably be the taking of a sworn oral deposition. In most malpractice cases, the involvement of the physician witness ends with a thorough deposition, if the parties agree to a settlement of the case. If a settlement is not reached, the physician will testify once more, this time in a formal courtroom trial.

At the trial, the direct examination of a medical witness is generally straightforward and uneventful, as noted in Chapter 2, especially when the physician and attorney have prepared carefully for the testifying. The cross-examination is another matter, as will be discussed in detail below.

Cross-Examining the Expert Witness

If the expert witness has delivered a flawless and impressive testimony, the opposing attorney will choose to make the cross-examination brief and uneventful. In most cases, however, the opposing attorney is obliged to do whatever is possible to diminish the contribution of the expert witness. The attorney can choose to question the following areas:

1.   The inadequate qualifications of the expert witness

2.   The limited data obtained by the expert witness

3.   The disagreement among physicians

4.   The scientific basis for the opinions

5.   Witness bias

Witness Qualification
"What makes you think you're an expert?"
Cross-examining attorneys can challenge an expert witness's qualifications to testify in a variety of ways. Note the following:

Q.   Doctor, you're board-certified in internal medicine, is that correct?

A.   That's correct.

Q.   You're not board-certified in endocrinology, are you?

A.   No, I'm not.

Q.   A board-certified physician in endocrinology specializes in treating diabetes, which is one of the medical issues in this case, isn't that true?

A.   Yes, that's true.

Q.   Since you are a specialist in internal medicine, wouldn't you defer to Dr. _____, who is board-certified in endocrinology?

a.   I have no problems with that.

It is unnecessary to defer to another medical specialist if you have a competent knowledge of the patient's medical condition and have the ability to diagnose and treat this disorder. A better response is

A. I regularly treat diabetic disorders in my specialty practice of internal medicine and have done so for more than 15 years. I am thoroughly familiar with this patient's medical condition and I do not think I need to defer to Dr. _____.

An expert's qualifications can also be questioned in the following manner:

Q. Doctor, you're from New York City, aren't you?

A. That's correct.

Q. How many days have you spent in our town altogether?

A. I arrived 3 days ago to review the patient's records and to prepare for this trial, so it's a total of 3 days.

Q. Are you testifying as to whether Dr. _____ met acceptable standards of medical practice when he treated the plaintiff?

A. Yes, I am.

Q. Isn't it a problem to testify about the acceptable standards of medical practice in this community when you just arrived three days ago?

a. Yes, it's a challenging problem, but I believe I can testify on this matter.

The jury will not be convinced simply because the expert has the confidence to testify. A more credible reply is

A. Although my office is in New York City, I have frequent opportunity to consult in smaller communities such as this one in various areas in the Northeast. The medical standards expected by you in this community should not, and I believe do not, differ much from the standards in any large metropolitan area.

Limited Data
"You mean you just saw the patient one time?"

Medical expert witnesses can be challenged with respect to the limited information they have in reaching their conclusions. Because they are often not the treating physician in the case, they have not had the same amount of direct contact with the patient, and this factor may be highlighted in the following inquiry:

Q. Doctor, when did you first examine the patient?

A. Three days ago, shortly after I arrived in town.

Q. How many times did you see the patient?

A. Just one time.

Q. You're aware that the patient has been under the care of Dr. _____ for the past 8 years, aren't you?

A. Yes, I am.

Q. Wouldn't you agree that a doctor who has examined a patient 30 times over 8 years knows that patient much better than a doctor who has seen the patient just once?

a. Yes.

A simple "Yes" answer practically eliminates the expert witness from contributing in this case because it suggests that the treating doctor, who knows the patient much better, has more valid opinions about the patient. To protect one's testimony, the reply should be

A. The treating doctor has more experience with the patient. Nonetheless, because of the vast research I have done on this case, including a review of all the patient's past medical records and work history, I am in a position to offer my expert opinion regarding the medical issues in this trial.

If the expert failed to respond, except with a simple "Yes," the defense attorney who retained the expert witness will probably ask questions on redirect examination to offset the impression left by the cross-examiner.

Q. Doctor, although you saw the patient only once, could you tell us again the extent of your investigation and evaluation in this case upon which you arrived at your expert opinion?

A. I have done vast research on this case, including a review of all the patient's past medical records and work history. Consequently, I believe I am in a position to offer my expert opinion regarding the medical issues in this trial.

Disagreement among Physicians:

"How can there be two different diagnoses for the same patient?"
Medical diagnoses are sometimes less precise than is generally perceived by the lay public. What one physician diagnoses as sciatica, another might label as lumbar radiculopathy. Because of the appearance of arbitrariness in medical diagnoses, the cross-examiner might attempt to emphasize the doubts that occur in the case.

Q. Besides the diagnosis of posttraumatic headaches, what alternative diagnoses did you consider for this patient?

A. I considered several other possibilities, such as migraine, muscle contracture headaches, cervical strain, or a functional, nonneurologic disorder.

Q. Is it likely that another physician can arrive at a different diagnosis than you did, such as migraine?

A. Yes, that's possible.

Q. And another doctor could have diagnosed her as having muscle contracture headaches, and yet another doctor could diagnose cervical strain?

A. Yes.

Q. In other words, four different doctors could come up with four different diagnoses for this patient, right?

a. That's right.

This response is inadequate and misleading. The jurors may incorrectly believe, based on the witness's answer, that doctors arrive at very different conclusions regarding a patient and that diagnoses are very subjective and unreliable. Consider this reply:

A. Four physicians may use different words to describe the patient, but they could agree that the person has suffered significant physical injuries as a result of the accident. The labels differ because the different doctors may place emphasis on different aspects of the person's medical condition. Studies have shown that clinical diagnoses among physicians are usually similar.

Scientific Basis for Opinions
"What's the scientific proof for your opinion?"

A physician who testifies about the presence of a medical disorder by identifying supportive laboratory tests typically has these conclusions accepted without challenge. However, an astute cross-examining attorney may insist that the medical expert fully explain the scientific bases for the diagnostic conclusions.

Q. Doctor, you testified that the cogwheel rigidity, bradykinesia, and rest tremor were indicative of the patient's Parkinson's disease. Do you have any scientific basis for reaching this conclusion?

a. Yes, in medical school and during my residency program, I was trained to interpret these findings in this manner.

This reply does not answer the attorney's question, and neither does the following:

a. I have many years of clinical experience with the signs and symptoms of Parkinson's disease, and I am confident of my diagnosis of this patient.

The attorney's serious inquiry into the scientific rationale for the diagnosis demands a more in-depth explanation of the findings.

A. Numerous studies have been conducted on patients with Parkinson's disease. Both laboratory and clinical studies have shown that the cogwheel rigidity, bradykinesia, and rest tremor correlate with insufficient dopamine in the striatum of a Parkinson disease patient's brain. An extensive body of research by Dr. _____ at the University of _____ Medical Center is the basis of some of my conclusions.

Although it is generally inadvisable to pontificate repeatedly while testifying, when faced with incisive questions, you should rise to the occasion and demonstrate the breadth of knowledge commensurate with your professional education and clinical experience. This display of medical authority will leave a positive impression in court as well as discourage the cross-examining attorney from further attempts to challenge your scientific credentials. Once you exhibit your level of expertise, the prudent attorney will retreat and avoid having you cause additional damage to the case.

Witness Bias
"Let's face it. Aren't you just a hired gun?'"
When all other forms of challenge fail, the cross-examiner will resort to what is essentially an ad hominem attack by suggesting that the expert witness is biased or that his or her opinion has been bought. Such an approach would proceed in the following way:

Q. Doctor, did you say that you're a specialist in treating diabetes?

A. Yes.

Q. And you say that you practice in this town?

A. Yes.

Q. Are you familiar with the defendant, Dr. _____?

A. Yes. I've known him professionally for more than 10 years, since I opened my practice here.

Q. Are you friends?

A. No. We're professional colleagues, but we're not friends.

Q. Have you ever testified in court before?

A. Yes.

Q. About how many times have you appeared in court?

A. Approximately five or six times.

Q. And when you appeared, was this for the patient or for the defense?

A. It was for the patient I was treating, not for the defense.

Q. Doctor, by your experiences in court, wouldn't you say that you tend to advocate for patients?

a. You could say that.

Q. Aren't you being paid by the patient to appear today?

a. Yes.

Q. Then, Doctor, you could be advocating for the patient today and against a colleague with whom you are not friendly, right?

a. That could be true.

The last three answers by the physician witness cast significant doubt on the objectivity of the testimony. Most doctors have testified in court because of their clinical association with their patients, and should respond:

A. I don't advocate for patients in court. I am here to testify as to the standard of medical care in this case.

Q. Aren't you being paid to testify by the patient today?

A. I am not being paid for my testimony. I am being paid for my expertise based on the time I spend in court.

Q. Doctor, you could be advocating for the patient today and against a colleague with whom you are not friendly, right?

A. No. I am not an advocate for one side, as an attorney must be. If I am an advocate, I am an advocate for the truth as I know it.

In scrutinizing apparent hired guns, the courts permit the questioning of an expert witness as to the annual income earned from testifying and also the frequency with which testimony is provided for certain sides, that is, for defense (e.g., insurance company) or plaintiff attorneys.

The Physician as the Defendant

Trial Preparation

There are few sentinel events in a physician's professional life that can be more emotionally devastating than being accused of medical malpractice. Physicians who find themselves in this crisis situation would benefit from reading *Doctors and the Law*, coauthored by a judge (Hiller B. Zobel) and a physician (Stephen N. Rous), which offers invaluable guidance to the physician charged with medical malpractice.[12]

Zobel and Rous advise the physician-defendant to have a close working relationship with the defense attorney who is provided by your malpractice insurance company to represent you in the lawsuit. The authors suggest a number of strategies, such as:

1. Do not respond to any letter or legal document pertaining to the malpractice claim. Let your lawyer handle all communications.

2. Do not contact your patient during the litigation, regardless of how much concern or regret you feel. Your expression of sincere sympathy can be interpreted as an admission of guilt. Nor should you call the patient out of anger or hurt, with a need to "set the record straight."

3. Keep a notebook to write down facts about the case that you recall, pertinent matters you want to discuss with your attorney, and technical publications that relate to the medical issues of your case. Be careful about relying on any such notes in depositions or in the courtroom because they could be designated as exhibits and open to scrutiny by the opposing side.

It is the defense attorney's responsibility to explain the legal aspects of the malpractice claim and the probable strategy of the plaintiff's attorney, so that the physician-defendant can clearly understand the legal principles involved in the case. Likewise, it is the physician's responsibility to explain the relevant medical issues (e.g., the management of the patient's care) in nontechnical language so that the attorney can understand the scientific facts of the case.[6] Because of the complexities of medical cases as well as legal procedures, the physician-defendant and the attorney must allocate substantial time and effort to preparation for the case.

In preparing for trial, the physician-defendant should make full disclosures to the defense attorney, citing the strengths along with the weaknesses in the case. The physician should assist the attorney by preparing a response to each charge of alleged wrongdoing, supported with documented medical knowledge. The physician must be forthcoming about any complaint against which it is difficult to defend, and if the physician is at fault, this should immediately be disclosed to the defense attorney, who may decide to settle the matter rather than attempt to defend the charges in court.

Many cases are settled by the opposing parties without going to court. However, many are not settled and proceed to trial. The physician-defendant must be present for all trial proceedings, and the recommendations made earlier for the physician witness in Chapter 2 regarding a court appearance apply to the physician-defendant as well. While sitting in court, the physician-defendant's clothing, posture, and demeanor are viewed constantly by the jurors. The physician must always appear serious and professional. Although it is impossible not to smile at times, physician-defendants should remember that they are on trial and that frequent laughter or grinning suggests that the charges are not being taken seriously. The physician should periodically look toward the jury but not glare at them or smile inappropriately. There is no room for emotional displays, such as anger at witnesses or dismay at the judge. Headshaking, scowling, and other gestures are to be avoided. The physician-defendant should keep busy by taking occasional notes that could assist the attorney.

The physician-defendant will eventually take the witness stand and provide valuable testimony in court. The suggestions for physician witnesses provided in Chapters 3 and 4 regarding direct and cross-examinations are applicable for the physician-defendant on the witness stand. The effectiveness of the physician-defendant in coping with the opposing attorney's cross-examination will play a pivotal role in determining the outcome of a malpractice trial. Your professional integrity and future are at stake, but it is not your responsibility to win the case as a witness. Your vigorous attempts at answering could be interpreted as self-righteousness or even guilty reactions. Simply answer what each question requires and nothing more. It is your attorney's responsibility to win the case.

Cross-Examining the Physician-Defendant

Physician-defendants will have their day in court, present their best explanation of the case, and then undergo a thorough cross-examination that will cover issues such as:

1. The acceptable standards of medical practice

2. The qualifications of the physician-defendant

3. Errors in the medical records

4. Higher medical standards

Acceptable Standards of Medical Practice
"You mean it's acceptable not to do a mammogram for a 39-year-old woman?"
Based on past court decisions, it would appear that as long as physicians follow an acceptable standard of medical practice, they will not

be held negligent. The following testimony typifies the questioning of the acceptability of a physician's medical performance:

Q. Doctor, when was the first time the patient told you about a lump in her breast?

A. That was on March 20, the day after her fortieth birthday.

Q. And when was the diagnosis of ductal breast carcinoma made?

A. The diagnosis was made on March 22, when she underwent breast mammography.

Q. Doctor, in your opinion, how long did the patient have this lump in her breast?

A. Based on the size and characteristics of the lump, I would say it was approximately 5 years.

Q. Is a breast mammogram routinely done with women under age 40?

A. No. Since the incidence of breast cancer in women under 40 is approximately 1 in 217, a breast mammogram is not routinely done for women in that age group. Women between 40 and 59 years of age, for whom the incidence of breast cancer is 1 in 26, should be considered for mammograms every 1–2 years depending on risk factors. Annual mammography is recommended after age 50.

Q. What is the incidence of breast cancer above age 40?

A. The incidence in women over 40 is 1 in 100, which is why we order breast mammograms routinely for them.

Q. I understand. Thank you, Doctor.

Usually this testimony will be sufficient to find the physician not guilty of medical negligence because the doctor adhered to the normal standards of medical care. However, exceptions have been made. For example, jurors may note that the incidence of breast cancer is low for women below 40 but that the mammogram is a simple and relatively inexpensive test. Thus, although the medical community may believe that no mammogram done before age 40 is acceptable practice, the lay community could conclude that the failure to provide this essential test in a timely manner constitutes negligence. This is rare but possible in a court of law.[5]

Qualifications of the Physician-Defendant
"Can any doctor treat diabetes?"

To convince the jury that acceptable standards of medical practice were not met, the cross-examining attorney may try to show that the physician-defendant had inadequate medical credentials, and ask the following questions:

Q. Doctor, you testified earlier that you are board-certified in family practice, is that right?

A. Yes, that's right.

Q. You're not board-certified in internal medicine, are you?

A. No, I'm not.

Q. You're not board-certified in endocrinology, are you?

A. No.

Q. Isn't it true that you have had less training in treating diabetes than a person trained in the specialties of internal medicine and endocrinology?

A. That's true.

Q. I acknowledge your general practice of medicine, but you haven't had anywhere near the hours of experience in treating diabetes as do specialists in internal medicine and endocrinology, isn't that right?

A. Although I haven't had as much experience as the specialists you mentioned, I do treat diabetics on a regular basis.

Q. But not nearly as much as the other specialists, right?

A. That's right.

Q. Don't most doctors refer diabetics to specialists rather than to family practitioners?

A. I don't know. That could be true.

Q. Then you would agree that the patient would have been better off being referred to a specialist than being treated by you, wouldn't you?

a. No, I disagree. I'm an experienced doctor and I know how to treat diabetes as well as anyone.

This defensive response would not be convincing with jurors. Instead, a response that emphasizes the generally accepted standards of medical practice would be better.

A. As a specialist in family practice, I am fully aware of the well-established guidelines for treating diabetes. I keep abreast of the current approaches and treatments, such as those practiced at the Joslin Center for Diabetes in Boston and recommended by the American Diabetic Association.

Some attorneys have considerable experience in the medicolegal area and may test the physician's credentials by a quiz on diabetes, such as the following:

Q. Doctor, can you tell me how insulin treatment doses are determined?

a. I begin with a standard dose of intermediate-acting insulin.

This brief and somewhat inadequate answer may be followed by even more pop quizzes. However, an attorney is less likely to pursue this line of questioning if the expert witness provides a clear and erudite answer to the question.

A. Insulin therapy is begun by administering a comparatively small dose of intermediate insulin such as NPH or lente insulin. This dose should be approximately 40% of the estimated daily insulin requirement for the patient. At ideal body weight, most patients require 30–50 units per day of exogenously administered highly purified insulin, whether given as a single preparation or in combination with another insulin preparation.

This response would demonstrate the physician's level of expertise, favorably impress the jury, and discourage the cross-examiner from further attempts to challenge the physician's medical knowledge.

Errors in the Medical Records
"Were you trained to make these kinds of errors, Doctor?"
When the complete medical records are available, it is easy for attorneys and their legal assistants to review the documents and discover various types of errors, usually of a clerical or typographical nature. These errors will be emphasized during court testimony and may imply

that adequate standards of medical practice were not maintained. The following questions may ensue:

Q. Doctor, when did you see the patient earlier this year?

A. It was on February 12.

Q. Could you tell us what your recent summary indicated as to the date?

A. (*after quickly reviewing the records*) It says February 21.

Q. Well, was it February 12 or February 21?

A. I'm sure it was February 12. That's what is indicated in the clinical records.

Q. Doctor, can you explain to us how the error took place?

A. It was evidently a typographical error that I missed when I proofread the summary.

Q. Your summary indicated that the patient had an appointment with you on July 5, is that correct?

A. (*again after reviewing the summary*) That's correct.

Q. The patient said he never saw you in July. Who is telling the truth?

A. (*after checking the clinical records*) He's right. We talked on the telephone on July 5 and I called in a prescription for him. We didn't have an actual office visit.

Q. Was he charged for an office visit because of that mistake?

A. (*another check of the files*) No. He wasn't charged.

Q. What did you prescribe for him on that day?

A. I prescribed Xanax, 0.5 milligram, to be taken twice a day for anxiety.

Q. Doctor, can you tell us what is typed in the patient's clinic records as to the prescription called in that day?

A. It says "Xanax, 5 milligrams, twice a day for anxiety."

Q. What would happen if your patient took 5 milligrams of Xanax twice a day?

a. He would be overly sedated and drowsy for several hours. That's too much Xanax, that's for sure.

Q. Doctor, weren't you trained to keep exact records and to write summaries that are accurate?

A. Yes.

Q. Are these mistakes standard or substandard levels of medical practice?

a. I guess I'd say they're substandard. I'm embarrassed to admit that.

Admitting to substandard practice is devastating in a trial in which the physician is being sued for negligence. There are better ways to respond to the above questions.

Q. What would happen if your patient took 5 milligrams of Xanax twice a day?

A. That could never happen. There is no Xanax in a 5-milligram form. The largest dose of Xanax available is 1 milligram. There was no mistake in the prescription I gave him; otherwise I would have heard from the pharmacist immediately. The prescription was incorrectly typed in his chart.

Q. Are these mistakes standard or substandard levels of medical practice?

A. There is no excuse for the clerical errors you noted. Fortunately, no such mistakes occurred in the delivery of medical care of this patient, which is my most important duty as a doctor.

The latter response acknowledges that mistakes were made of a clerical nature and refocuses the concern toward the appropriate medical care of the patient.

Higher Medical Standards
"Isn't it wise to use the best tests available?"

A cross-examination that identifies better ways of diagnosing or treating a patient will suggest that an appropriate level of medical practice was not pursued. Note the following questions:

Q. Doctor, please tell us how you arrived at your diagnosis of this patient.

A. In addition to my medical examination of him, I ordered an MRI scan of the brain, as well as a PSVER, or pattern shift visual evoked response.

Q. In retrospect, what other tests could you have requested to help in diagnosing this patient?

A. Well, I could have asked for an SER, or somatosensory evoked response, and a cerebrospinal fluid evaluation. This would have indicated a demyelinating disorder, such as multiple sclerosis.

Q. Can you name any other diagnostic procedures that are used in cases like this?

A. Yes, sometimes a BAER, or brainstem auditory evoked response, is done. On other occasions a CT scan is ordered.

Q. Do you know if BAER studies and CT scans are done at the University Medical Center?

A. Yes. I'm sure they do those tests there.

Q. Why didn't you request that those tests be done on the patient?

a. Well, those are expensive tests and I didn't think the added costs were warranted. He's in a managed care program that is pretty frugal when it comes to expensive diagnostic tests.

Q. But wouldn't those tests have given additional information about his condition?

a. Yes.

The latter two answers will imply that a clinical decision was made for economic, not medical, reasons and that the patient's health care was compromised. Better responses would be

Q. Why didn't you request that those tests be done on the patient?

A. For the diagnosis of multiple sclerosis, the routine tests are an MRI and a PSVER, and those were obtained immediately. The CT scans and BAER are less specific and sensitive and are not indicated and are rarely requested in cases like this.

Q. But wouldn't those tests have given additional information about the patient?

A. The additional tests might have simply been redundant. As I testified earlier, the tests I ordered are the usual tests requested in this kind of case, and I had complete information to reach a diagnosis.

If a physician performs the usual medical tests for a particular condition, no medical negligence has been committed. The physician is not judged by the highest standard of care, such as the ordering of multiple tests that might be done at a teaching hospital.

Closing Arguments

Medical malpractice suits arise when it is alleged that (1) the physician had a duty to care for the plaintiff, (2) the physician failed in the duty to care, (3) the failure to care resulted in damage to the plaintiff, and (4) the damage can be measured for monetary compensation. In medical malpractice cases, a key role is played by a physician expert witness who will help to define the acceptable standards of medical practice and show that medical negligence occurred when the physician's failure in the duty to care led to significant damages to the plaintiff.

Physicians who testify as expert witnesses in medical malpractice cases provide an invaluable service, because their testimony will help to exonerate the physician whose professional conduct meets the acceptable standard of medical care or will hold negligent physicians accountable for their substandard performance.

Physicians who are defendants in a medical malpractice case are advised to work cooperatively with the insurance company's attorney who will represent them in the litigation, to educate the attorney about the medical issues in the case, and to follow the advice and direction from the attorney. Physician-defendants on the witness stand have the enormous challenge of coping with not only complex medicolegal questions, but with direct assaults on their professional competence and integrity.

This chapter provided samples of challenging cross-examinations for medical expert witnesses as well as for physician-defendants. Because of the high stakes usually involved in medical malpractice cases, both types of witnesses can expect a vigorous cross-examination, but they can provide effective testimony when they are aware of the legal issues involved in medical negligence litigation and the kinds of tactics employed by opposing attorneys. A thumbnail summary on medical malpractice is found in Appendix D.

References

1. Jamieson EL, Seaman B. The frontiers of medicine. *Time* 1996;148(14): 1–86.
2. Rice B. Where doctors get sued the most. *Med Econ* 1995; 14(2):98–110.
3. Mason JK. *Forensic Medicine for Lawyers*. Bristol, England: Wright & Sons, 1978.
4. Dunn JD. Medical Testimony: Physician as Witness. In American College of Legal Medicine (ed), *Legal Medicine: Legal Dynamics of Medical Encounters* (2nd ed). St. Louis: Mosby–Year Book, 1991;535–539.
5. Quimby CW. General Considerations of Medical Testimony. In AE James (ed), *Legal Medicine: With Special Reference to Diagnostic Imaging*. Baltimore: Urban & Schwarzenberg, 1980;49–61.
6. McGugin DE. Preparation of the Physician for Trial. In AE James (ed), *Legal Medicine: With Special Reference to Diagnostic Imaging*. Baltimore: Urban & Schwarzenberg, 1980;63–74.
7. Curran WJ. *Tracy's The Doctor as a Witness*. Philadelphia: Saunders, 1965.
8. Texas Rev Civil Stat 4590, §14.01 (1990 suppl).
9. Block B. Evolving legal standards for the admissibility of scientific evidence. *Science* 1988;239:1508–1512.
10. Komins JI, Komins DJ. The expert witness: the whole truth and nothing but . . . *Obstet Gynecol Surv* 1996;51:265–266.
11. Vevaina JR, Finz LL. The Expert Witness in Medical Malpractice Litigation. In JR Vevaina, RC Bone, E Kassoff (eds), *Legal Aspects of Medicine*. New York: Springer-Verlag, 1989;33–38.
12. Zobel HB, Rous SN. *Doctors and the Law*. New York: WW Norton, 1993.

8

Medicolegal Issues for Medical and Surgical Specialties

Medical practice today consists of a vast complex of specializations. There are 23 sanctioned American specialty boards (Table 8-1), and many medical societies and organizations break down further into numerous self-designated practice specialties (Table 8-2).

Because the previous chapters of this book were broadly oriented, it is fitting to provide some specific information and advice for the various medical specialists. Not all the medical specialties will be covered in this chapter; only those types of medical, surgical, and ancillary services that are most frequently involved in legal activity will be discussed, with attention given to the legal issues and proceedings involved with these specialties.

It should be realized that from 60% to 80% of all trial level cases in American courts and administrative tribunals involve medical factual issues.[1] Neurologic and orthopedic cases lead all other specialties in the volume of work in the courts of the United States.[2,3] This chapter addresses the medicolegal issues in obstetrics/gynecology, pediatrics, general practice, family practice, internal medicine, general surgery, orthopedics, physiatry, neurology, plastic and reconstructive surgery, psychiatry, pathology, and radiology.

Obstetrics/Gynecology and Pediatrics

Because of their responsibilities in the care of mothers and babies, the specialists in obstetrics and pediatrics have been involved in major

Table 8-1. American Specialty Boards

American Board of Allergy and Immunology

American Board of Anesthesiology

American Board of Colon and Rectal Surgery

American Board of Dermatology

American Board of Emergency Medicine

American Board of Family Practice

American Board of Internal Medicine

American Board of Neurological Surgery

American Board of Nuclear Medicine

American Board of Obstetrics and Gynecology

American Board of Ophthalmology

American Board of Orthopaedic Surgery

American Board of Otolaryngology

American Board of Pathology

American Board of Pediatrics

American Board of Physical Medicine and Rehabilitation

American Board of Plastic Surgery

American Board of Preventive Medicine

American Board of Psychiatry and Neurology

American Board of Radiology

American Board of Surgery

American Board of Thoracic Surgery

American Board of Urology

---

medicolegal litigation, primarily medical malpractice cases. The transcendent objective of obstetrics is that every pregnancy culminates in a healthy mother and a healthy baby. While the large majority of mothers and babies conclude the course of pregnancy, labor, and puerperium in a healthy physical and mental state, contemporary obstetrics has to contend with a higher rate of teenage pregnancies, the availability of abused substances, including legal and illicit drugs, and the advent of new life-saving neonatal technologies, along with the concomitant high-risk pregnancies, drug-dependent mothers, and premature babies that threaten a healthy birth experience.

Table 8-2. Self-Designated Practice Specialties

Abdominal Surgery

Addiction Medicine

Addiction Psychiatry

Adolescent Medicine

Adult Reconstructive Orthopedics

Aerospace Medicine

Allergy

Allergy and Immunology

Allergy/Immunology, Diagnostic
    Laboratory Immunology

Anatomic/Clinical Pathology

Anatomic Pathology

Anesthesiology

Blood Banking/Transfusion
    Medicine

Cardiac Electrophysiology

Cardiovascular Diseases

Cardiovascular Surgery

Chemical Pharmacology

Child and Adolescent Psychiatry

Child Neurology

Clinical Biochemical Genetics

Clinical Cytogenetics

Clinical Genetics

Clinical Molecular Genetics

Clinical Neurophysiology

Clinical Pathology

Clinical Pharmacology

Cytopathology

Colon and Rectal Surgery

Critical Care Medicine
    (Anesthesiology)

Critical Care Medicine (Internal
    Medicine)

Critical Care Medicine
    (Neurologic Surgery)

Critical Care Medicine (Obstetrics
    and Gynecology)

Critical Care Medicine (Pediatric)

Critical Care Medicine (Surgery)

Dermatologic Immunology, Diag-
    nostic Laboratory Immunology

Dermatology

Dermatopathology

Diabetes

Diagnostic Laboratory Immunology
    (Internal Medicine)

Diaganostic Laboratory
    Immunology (Pediatrics)

Diagnostic Radiology

Emergency Medicine

Endocrinology, Diabetes
    and Metabolism

Facial Plastic Surgery

Family Practice

Forensic Pathology

Forensic Psychiatry

Gastroenterology

General Practice

General Preventive Medicine

General Surgery

Geriatric Medicine (Family Practice)

Geriatric Medicine (Internal
    Medicine)

Geriatric Psychiatry

Gynecological Oncology

Gynecology

Hand Surgery (Orthopedic Surgery)

Hand Surgery (Plastic Surgery)

Table 8-2. continued

Hand Surgery (Surgery)	Orthopedic Surgery
Head and Neck Surgery	Orthopedic Surgery of the Spine
Hematology (Internal Medicine)	Orthopedic Trauma
Hematology (Pathology)	Other Specialty
Hepatology	Otolaryngology
Immunology	Otology
Immunopathology	Pain Management (Anesthesiology)
Infectious Diseases	Pediatric Allergy
Internal Medicine	Pediatric Cardiology
Legal Medicine	Pediatric Emergency Medicine
Maternal and Fetal Medicine	Pediatric Endocrinology
Medical Genetics	Pediatric Gastroenterology
Medical Microbiology	Pediatric Hematology-Oncology
Medical Oncology	Pediatric Infectious Diseases
Medical Toxicology (Emergency Medicine)	Pediatric Nephrology
	Pediatric Orthopedics
Medical Toxicology (Pediatrics)	Pediatric Otolaryngology
Medical Toxicology (Preventive Medicine)	Pediatric Pathology
	Pediatric Pulmonology
Musculoskeletal Oncology	Pediatric Radiology
Neonatal-Perinatal Medicine	Pediatric Rheumatology
Nephrology	Pediatric Surgery
Neurologic Surgery	Pediatric Surgery (Neurology)
Neurology	Pediatric Urology
Neuropathology	Pediatrics
Neuroradiology	Physical Medicine and Rehabilitation
Nuclear Medicine	Plastic Surgery
Nuclear Radiology	Psychiatry
Nutrition	Psychoanalysis
Obstetrics	Public Health
Obstetrics and Gynecology	Pulmonary Disease
Occupational Medicine	Radiation Oncology
Ophthalmology	Radioisotopic Pathology
Orthopedic Sports Medicine (Orthopedic Surgery)	

Radiologic Physics	Sports Medicine (Pediatrics)
Radiology	Thoracic Surgery
Reproductive Endocrinology	Traumatic Surgery
Rheumatology	Undersea Medicine
Sports Medicine (Emergency Medicine)	Unspecified
	Urologic Surgery
Sports Medicine (Family Practice)	Vascular and Interventional Radiology
Sports Medicine (Internal Medicine)	Vascular Surgery

At all times of pregnancy, the obstetrician may encounter various anomalies involving the mother or fetus, such as spontaneous or intentional abortion, premature labor, and ectopic pregnancy. Problems may also arise during labor including dystocia, injuries to the birth canal, and abnormalities of the third stage of labor. During the puerperium the obstetrician may be faced with infections, hematomas, and thromboembolic disease.

The fetus may sustain injuries during pregnancy and labor, such as fetal distress, prolapse of the umbilical cord, and cerebral hemorrhage. There may be malformations of the fetus, for example, chromosome anomalies, spina bifida, or congenital heart disease. Other medical conditions of the newborn include prematurity, respiratory distress, and substance dependence.

The above myriad (and hardly complete) list of disorders and abnormalities can potentially be interpreted as a bad result or medical negligence and thus the obstetrician is at risk for a malpractice complaint. The severity of the mother's or baby's disability will be predictive of the monetary compensation for the plaintiff, and when birth-related injury cases are resolved, medical claims that exceed $1 million are not uncommon. The escalating rise in medical negligence claims against obstetricians, and other physicians as well, has led to a trend toward defensive medical practice.[4] Even when tests have known limited clinical value, they may be ordered for medicolegal reasons, especially if a physician fears potential litigation.

An obstetrician also has extensive training in gynecology, which is the medical specialty that deals with the physiology and pathology of the female reproductive organs in the nonpregnant state. Because of the increased malpractice risks inherent in obstetrics, many of today's ob-gyn specialists limit their practice to gynecology. However, gynecologists also encounter medicolegal issues such as failed sterilization, contraceptive problems, complications of abortions and hysterectomies, and misdiagnoses of cancer.[5]

Specialists in pediatrics, as well as obstetricians, are at risk for a malpractice claim in cases of neonatal complications, such as asphyxia, intracranial hemorrhage, infections, and seizures. Child anomalies such as cerebral palsy, mental retardation, and developmental disorders may be interpreted by plaintiffs to be the result of negligence on the part of the obstetrician and sometimes the pediatrician. Childhood illnesses such as bronchitis and pneumonia, vomiting and diarrhea, high fevers, and congenital heart disease pose serious threats to babies, and their complications may develop into serious medicolegal issues for the pediatrician.

The price tag for pediatric negligence claims skyrockets when the illness results in brain damage and mental retardation. In these cases, claims alleging brain damage can be made up to 18 or 21 years after the incident, depending on the specific jurisdiction where the claim is made. The law provides a broad statute of limitations for injured children, with legal proceedings hampered by the loss of medical evidence and records and even by the departure or death of parties involved in the case.[5]

In a survey of 255 pediatricians in Pennsylvania, nearly one-half provided expert testimony in medical malpractice cases at some time.[6] However, these physicians were also selective about their involvement as expert witnesses, as 96 (76%) had refused to give testimony at some time for various reasons, such as not believing there was a legitimate malpractice case, concerns about the attorney's motions, and beliefs that they were not qualified experts for the case.

Pediatricians are also involved in the legal system in personal injury cases, such as when a child is injured in a traffic accident. Recent involvement in family courts have increased because of the greater number of reported incidents of child abuse and neglect, as well as in cases of substance abuse and juvenile criminal behaviors.

Obstetrician/gynecologists and pediatricians who work in hospital settings often operate within urgent and tight time constraints. In the courtroom, the opposing attorney wants to emphasize the limited time factor to show that there was a rush to judgment or to discredit the work done.

Q. If you had more time and information in your assessment of this case, wouldn't that cause you to change your opinion?

a. Possibly.

One never knows if more time and information would result in a change of opinion, but to admit that you did not have enough time would not be excusable in most jurors' minds. When you believe that you had adequate time and information to make a decision, then you should state

A. Although time was limited when I saw the patient, I had sufficient information to reach a firm diagnosis. Otherwise, I would have insisted on more time or informed the patient that I could not reach a decision on the matter.

General Practice, Family Practice, and Internal Medicine

Physicians in general practice, family practice, and internal medicine have one thing in common: They treat a full range of diseases and symptomatic complaints that arise in their medical practices. Because of the broad scope of their work, many of these primary care physicians, especially the general and family practitioners, see themselves as "jacks of all trades" and not as "experts" from the usual medical standpoint with regard to a particular disease. However, from the legal standpoint these generalists are indeed experts who bring to legal disputes knowledge and experience that are beyond the ken of the average layperson, and they have the right, as well as the duty, to appear as expert witnesses in a court of law.

General practice, family practice, and internal medicine physicians will occasionally be called as witnesses in a personal injury case as a result of being the plaintiff's primary treating physician. (Sometimes they may be bypassed if the patient was also referred to a specialist, such as an orthopedic surgeon.) Unlike ordinary lay witnesses who can only testify as to what they observed, a treating physician is accorded a wide latitude when testifying as a witness. For example, a treating physician can report the symptoms and suffering reported by the patient, as such statements are not barred by the hearsay rule.[7] Treating physicians can provide diagnoses and prognoses, and also can render an opinion about whether or not the patient is malingering.

The rendering of an opinion regarding the causal relation between trauma and disease, such as a heart condition, stroke, or cancer, is one of the troublesome questions facing a treating physician. In this regard, physicians must familiarize themselves with the legal concepts of causation, in contrast to medical concepts of causation. In law, *a causal relationship is established if an injury aggravates, hastens, or precipitates a disease or condition*,[8] and it is not essential that the trauma is an etiologic cause. The treating doctor must take a complete history from the patient and keep well-documented records because the causation issues that are addressed at the time of the trial will require a thorough grasp of all possible relevant factors. If the treating physician has not conducted a thorough investigation of the case, then an opinion about causation should not be rendered.

Because the exact etiology in certain cases may not be crystal clear, the opposing counsel will try to extract damaging testimony from the physician on the witness stand. For example, the cross-examining attorney may ask,

Q. Doctor, is it your speculation that the car accident caused the patient's heart attack?

a. Yes.

The key word is "speculation," and the significance of the question is that guessing is implied. If the physician is certain to a reasonable medical probability, that is, 51% sure, the response should be

A. No. There is no speculation or guessing here. My opinion, based on a reasonable medical certainty, is that the car accident caused the patient's heart attack.

Because of the nature of their medical practice, physicians in general practice, family practice, and internal medicine may find themselves in a greater variety of legal hearings than most specialists. In addition to the more common personal injury and workers' compensation cases, they may be asked for their medical opinions in domestic matters (e.g., spousal abuse), life insurance issues, motor vehicle licensing questions, and criminal cases. Additionally, these physicians may be called in to will contests when they are asked for their opinion regarding the mental competence of a person who died leaving the will in question. This is not a question on which only a psychiatrist's opinion is admissible into evidence. Physicians should gain some familiarity with such legal problems involved in their patients' cases and the relevance of the medical testimony to those issues.

General practice, family practice, and internal medicine physicians must also contend with medical malpractice claims against them. The notion that personal physicians are relatively immune from malpractice suits because of their close relationship with patients is no longer valid. In recent years, over one-third of general and family physicians have incurred malpractice claims in their careers.[9]

At the time of the courtroom appearance, primary care physicians will be relieved to learn that, as personal physicians, they are generally well-received by the lay jurors.[2] Opposing attorneys hesitate to attack "the family doctor," the "Marcus Welby" of the community. Primary care physicians could encounter difficulties in court if they appear to offer an opinion outside of their competence and in the realm of a subspecialist. Attorneys may discredit the generalist as not qualified to render certain opinions, but the physician will be on firm foundations when providing clearly reasoned and well-documented evidence. Testimony by primary care physicians is especially relevant in medical malpractice cases involving a peer, as they are in the best position to judge if the management and treatment by a fellow general practitioner, family physician, or internist met the standard of care in the community.[10]

General Surgery

Like the primary care practitioners discussed in the previous sections, general surgeons may become involved medicolegally in a variety of situations from medical malpractice to personal injury. Physicians in general surgery are generally not known to be among the high-risk specialists in terms of malpractice charges, but the number of claims they have encountered has increased in recent years. A frequent charge is inadequate experience, that is, surgeons without sufficient skills should not undertake certain procedures, such as recently developed "micro" and "scopic" techniques not available to older surgeons during their residencies. It is difficult to defend against the claim of inadequate experience if the general surgeon performs a certain operation only a few times a year.[11] However, in emergency situations general surgeons are expected

to manage various problems and do not always have the luxury of referring the patient to an available experienced subspecialist.

Previous malpractice litigation has led to the articulation of a principle referred to as "the captain of the ship" doctrine, which states that
the surgeon in charge is responsible for the staff with whom the surgeon is working, including residents, interns, and even the anesthesi-
ologist.[12] Thus, a malpractice claim against a surgeon can extend to
medical care given at night or during the weekend when the surgeon
is off-duty. Surgeons must therefore exercise careful management of
and communications with the surgical team members to insure that
proper patient care is exercised at all times.

Errors in diagnosis are among the common claims against general
surgeons. Missed diagnoses, such as perforated peptic ulcers and acute
appendicitis, may occur. Even though an erroneous conclusion was
reached, these charges may be defensible if a proper history was taken
and a thorough examination was performed.

The most widely reported type of malpractice case against general
surgeons involves the failure to diagnose breast cancer.[11] The surgeon
who does not consider an adequate biopsy or other tests necessary for
a vague ill-defined area of thickening in the breast will be in serious
legal difficulty if the mass subsequently proves to be a carcinoma.
Because of the availability of methods such as mammography and fine
needle aspiration, it is difficult to mount a defense against the failure
to evaluate breast lumps thoroughly.

Surgeons should document the basis for surgical decisions and keep
complete operative notes and records. With regard to postoperative visits, both physical findings as well as subjective complaints should be
detailed. Surgeons should be aware that the legal system desires objective signs of disease and injury whenever possible and practicable.
Thus, if a surgical case is likely to have medicolegal consequences, it
may be prudent to request certain diagnostic tests so that objective evidence may be available, not only for the purpose of defensive medicine,
but also for the sake of the patient, the courts, and all those involved.

In the event that they are asked to serve as an expert witness in a surgical malpractice case, surgeons should be abreast of the currently
acceptable and nonacceptable procedures in surgery in order to establish the standard of care. They should familiarize themselves with the
methods of measuring physical disability and estimating prognoses.
Opinions on prognoses should not be overly optimistic, as when clinicians reassure their anxious patients, nor overly pessimistic, as may be
wanted by some aggressive plaintiff lawyers for legal advantages.

As is the case with other physicians, one of the most critical medicolegal issues pertains to the cause of the patient's health condition. For surgeons, the legal issue is to determine if trauma, whether single, continuous, or cumulative over a period of time, caused or aggravated the problem (e.g., pain). The requirements of causation in law must be clearly understood,[8] or one should ask the attorney to explain the requirements before forming an opinion. Consider the following question:

Q. Doctor, with all the many possible causes of abdominal pain, isn't it difficult to be certain about the cause of this woman's abdominal pain?

a. Yes. It is.

Agreeing with the question is not altogether wrong, because it is often difficult to identify the precise cause of a person's abdominal pain. However, without further explanation, the jurors can mistakenly conclude that the witness is undecided about the cause of the patient's pain. A clearer answer would be

A. Indeed the diagnosis of abdominal pain is not a simple one. I fully considered all of the possible causes you mentioned, such as ulcers, diverticulitis, endometriosis, and stress, and it is my opinion that the irritable bowel syndrome from the car accident was the sole cause of the abdominal pain she has had in the past year.

Orthopedic Surgery, Physical Rehabilitation/Sports Medicine, Neurology, and Neurosurgery

The specialists in orthopedic surgery, physical rehabilitation/sports medicine, neurology, and neurosurgery, are grouped together because of their common experience with physical trauma cases that become inextricably involved in the medicolegal system, usually in the form of personal injury lawsuits or workers' compensation claims. Because of the legal entanglements of their posttrauma cases, the specialists in this category should possess as clear an understanding as possible of how the person was injured because the manner of the occurrence and the physics of the trauma itself will be important in the explanation of the alleged injuries. In a motor vehicle accident case, the relevant factors include

- The date, time, and environmental conditions (e.g., daylight, weather, traffic)

- The type of impact (e.g., rear-end, head-on, broadside), the speed of the vehicles involved, and damage to the vehicles

- Where the patient was seated in the automobile, the use and type of seat restraints (e.g., lap belt, shoulder belt, air bag)

- The objects the patient struck within the car at impact (e.g., dashboard, windshield, head restraints)

- Whether there was a head injury (e.g., loss of consciousness, scalp laceration, bruising, bleeding)

- The police and ambulance reports at the scene, especially medic assessments of Glasgow Coma Scale score, vital signs, and injuries sustained

- Whether the patient was treated medically at the scene and if the injured person was taken by ambulance, by others, or drove to an emergency room

- The emergency room report, including diagnoses, treatment, and recommendations

- When and where the injured person was seen in follow-up by a physician or other health care providers

In industrial injury cases, the physician should ascertain the following:

- The date, time, place, and work environment

- The details of how the accident occurred (e.g., fall from scaffold, electrocution, explosion)

- The areas of the body traumatized and the extent of the injuries

- When and how the injuries were treated and whether emergency medical care and an ambulance were provided (similar details as noted in the previous personal injury section)

- The first time the patient received medical care and by whom

- Any unusual hazards or risks at the job site (e.g., exposed electrical wires, no hard hat or steel-toed shoes)

In addition to a thorough history, the physician should be able to describe the mechanism of the injury—the type of force that was exerted on the back resulting in a herniated disc, for example. For the purpose of testifying, the physician witness should have educational aids (e.g., anatomic drawings or models) to explain the physical injury. Detailed records of the physical examination will help to explain how diagnoses were confirmed. Physicians need to explain subjective complaints, such as pain, and objective signs, such as magnetic resonance imaging (MRI) results. The review of previous medical examinations and tests is also essential.

The physician will be asked to assess the patient's levels of functioning and should be able to estimate the degree of the disability, often expressed in percentages, and its duration, whether temporary or permanent, using the *AMA Guides to the Evaluation of Permanent Impairment*.[13] In these cases, legal arguments will often revolve around pre-existing medical conditions versus recent injuries. Recovery for the plaintiff will be allowed when the trauma aggravates a pre-existing condition, but serious questions will also arise whether the trauma had anything to do with the exacerbation of previous symptoms. An issue of concern with trauma cases is the question of prognosis because some of these patients with spinal or head injuries are likely to be seriously injured, require long periods of treatment, and incur long-term disability residuals of varying degrees. The pain and suffering of the plaintiff will also be important elements in the assessment of damages, particularly in personal injury tort cases, and the physician must be prepared to offer evidence on this issue.

Physicians must be prepared for some jurisdictional disputes between their specialty and others. A common area of dispute is the interpretation of skeletal x-ray films, computed tomographic (CT) scans, and MRI scans. A cross-examining lawyer may suggest,

Q. Doctor, isn't the interpretation of imaging results within the expertise of a radiologist rather than your field?

a. That's true.

The appropriate reply by an orthopedist, physiatrist, or neurologic specialist is

A. There is an overlap between my specialty and that of radiology. Physicians in my specialty are qualified in the specialized area of interpreting imaging results. Moreover, with my clinical experience and my knowledge of this particular patient, I am eminently qualified to form an opinion about the CT scan results.

The specialty of orthopedic surgery consists of the treatment of the spine, bones, joints, and surrounding soft tissues. Because a large number of accidental injuries involve these physical structures, the orthopedist is the physician most involved in medicolegal activity such as testifying in court or before workers' compensation hearing boards.

The types of orthopedic problems are many and varied, and the more common legal cases involve trauma of the back and neck. The largest group of spinal injury patients are those with low back complaints, either with or without lumbar disc trauma. Objective findings of a spinal injury, such as lacerations and fractures, will be important for medical and legal reasons. In certain cases, an MRI study of the spine to confirm a disc injury may be advisable, even though the clinical findings on examination seem adequate to the orthopedist.

The second largest group of patients with spine injuries are those with cervical spine trauma. The majority of these cases result from rear-end traffic collisions with sequelae that have been termed *whiplash* injuries. Because whiplash has no specific medical definition, the term should be avoided in medical reports, hearings, depositions, and trials. If used while on the witness stand, the term *whiplash*, because of its controversial history, may provoke an extensive cross-examination.[2]

With respect to medical malpractice claims, the orthopedic surgeon represents one of the high-risk specialties. Although untoward surgical results are not necessarily proof of malpractice, orthopedists are sued for surgical complications, such as infection, which is a common risk factor, especially when a bone has pierced the skin. Orthopedists are at risk in spinal surgeries that could lead to chronic pain or paralysis. Tight casts with related nerve damage have resulted in malpractice suits, although this is less of a problem with modern improvements in casting and techniques. As with other specialties, in order for an orthopedic malpractice claim to be upheld, the plaintiff must prove violations of the standard of care or a lack of informed consent.[14]

In recent years, trauma injury patients frequently have been referred to physiatrists, who are specialists in physical medicine and rehabilitation and also sports medicine. Physiatrists treat patients with neck and back injuries, direct physical therapy regimens, and perform electrodiagnostic studies, namely electromyographic (EMG) and nerve conduction studies. Either independently or with orthopedic colleagues, certain physiatrists have specialized in sports medicine and treat athletes and their sports-related trauma. Because of the increasing referrals of nonsurgical orthopedic injuries to physical medicine specialists, many of the medicolegal cases previously facing orthopedic surgeons now become the domain of the physiatrist, including issues regarding causation, treatment, and prognosis of neck and back injuries.

The specialists in *neurology* and *neurosurgery* perform various roles in today's legal processes. They provide medical opinions to attorneys and courts to help resolve disputes relating to neurologic disease or injury. They develop criteria for the management of neurologic patients that are used as legal standards of care. They provide data to public officials and legislators that are used in drafting laws regarding such matters as motor vehicle driving and brain death.[15]

The most frequent types of medicolegal cases in which neurologists and neurosurgeons become involved are injuries to the head, neck, and back. Traumatic head injuries are unfortunately a common occurrence in traffic and industrial accidents, requiring the assessment and treatment of concussion, brain injury, and post-traumatic epilepsy. Brain damage and paralysis result in some of the highest lawsuit settlements in our courts, placing neurologists and neurosurgeons in the midst of highly contested litigations. While the severe brain injury cases result in maximum monetary awards, the most contentious medicolegal disputes arise in cases of mild head injury and claims of a postconcussive syndrome, with difficult-to-document neurobehavioral and psychoemotional dysfunction.[16]

Whereas the neurologic clinician focuses on diagnosis, treatment, and rehabilitation, the neurologic expert in the medicolegal setting evaluates patients long after an injury, focusing less on therapy and more on the degree of permanent disability to determine appropriate monetary compensation. Furthermore, in medicolegal practice, neurologists and neurosurgeons must account for nonneurologic factors, such as symptom magnification and compensation neurosis, that are not ordinarily emphasized in their everyday clinical work. These neurologic experts must carefully assess the patient's subjective reports, which are affected not only by the prospects of financial gain but also by brain injury that may prevent patients from accurately perceiving their own dysfunctions.[17]

When medicolegal cases are involved, neurologic specialists should perform comprehensive diagnostic procedures to confirm clinical impressions, including pertinent brain and spinal CT and MRI scans, electroencephalograms (EEGs), nerve conduction studies, and somatosensory evoked responses (SERs). The failure to conduct adequate diagnostic procedures can come under sharp criticism during cross-examination.

The testimony of a neurologist and neurosurgeon involves a thorough description of the neurologic injury and impairment. They will testify as to any direct relation between a head injury and sequelae such as headaches and cognitive impairment. On occasion, they must comment on the less direct relation between head injury and the onset of depression or multiple sclerosis.

In recent years, neurologists have been called on to address alleged injuries to the nervous system from neurotoxins. Referred to as *toxic torts*, these medicolegal cases are among the most controversial in the courts today and include the well-publicized ailments from exposure to Agent Orange, the claims of carcinogenic and neurologic disorders from electromagnetic field radiation, and possible autoimmune disorders from silicone breast implants.[18]

Malpractice claims against neurologic specialists are varied. Some of the cases involve delayed diagnoses, such as the finding of a meningioma or a subdural or epidural hematoma after trauma. Some involve missed diagnoses, such as not identifying meningitis, peripheral nerve injuries, or a subarachnoid hemorrhage despite classic symptoms. The failure to prevent a disorder (e.g., a cerebrovascular accident) and the inadequate or delayed treatment of hemorrhages are also objects of malpractice claims for these practitioners. The neurosurgeon shares the same risk patterns as other surgeons, but because of the devastating effects of brain and spinal mishaps, they often face malpractice claims of major proportions.

Plastic and Reconstructive Surgery

For years, specialists in plastic and reconstructive surgery have been among the physicians who encounter the greatest number of malpractice complaints. With today's plastic surgeons aggressively advertising their work in cosmetic procedures on television and the print media, plastic surgery cases will continue to be among the most common malpractice lawsuits in the future.[19] Handsome monetary compensation will be awarded not only for the physical scars and unfavorable surgical results, but patients also will be compensated for postoperative pain and emotional scars as well.

More than most medical specialists, plastic surgeons are aware that they must never promise or guarantee particular results. The public has high expectations, sometimes unrealistically, of what cosmetic surgery can produce, and an unhappy patient can easily become a vengeful plaintiff. Photographs of the patient before and after surgery are basic procedures, as well as accurate descriptions of the patient's physical conditions, as the prime issue in plastic surgery cases revolves around the surgical outcome.

Cosmetic and reconstructive surgeons are required to know the impact of surgical procedures, medications, and surgery-related products on their patients. One of the most publicized medical malpractice issues has involved product liability, with the use of silicone implants reportedly causing systemic disease and resulting in multimillion-dollar settlements.[20,21] Experienced and competent plastic surgeons must be willing to step forward to testify in these complex and controversial lawsuits rather than leave the medicolegal explanations to so-called "suitcase doctors" and "crossover specialists."

Plastic surgeons are also involved in personal injury cases in which they are asked if future operations can repair a patient's scars. Defense attorneys hope for optimal predictions so that monetary damages can be reduced in these tort cases. The witness must be careful in answering this important question. Cosmetic surgical outcomes are difficult to predict, except with a general estimate of the results, and the plastic surgeon must resist the lawyer's or judge's request for a more precise prognosis.

Psychiatry

Physician witnesses offer their professional knowledge in a variety of legal venues, and the specialists in psychiatry are a prime example.[22] Psychiatric experts are probably most visible when they testify regarding the insanity/responsibility issue in high-profile criminal cases, such as the trial of John Hinckley, who shot former President Ronald Reagan in 1981. Psychiatric testimony is essential with today's burgeoning personal injury lawsuits that claim physical as well as emotional sequelae from traffic accidents, particularly those involving a postconcussion syndrome and chronic pain. Psychiatrists are needed to determine mental competency in civil proceedings (e.g., will contests) and in commercial litigation. Divorce and child custody hearings also demand psychiatric evaluations to resolve often bitter marital dissolutions. The expertise of psychiatrists may have an impact on the court process itself when they assist in jury selection or when they testify as to the fallibility of eyewitnesses.

Although psychiatrists remain one of the most frequently employed medical witnesses in the jurisprudence system, they are also among the most maligned. Several reasons are apparent for the widespread skepticism toward psychiatry in the courtroom. First, it is not uncommon for experienced and respected psychiatrists to contradict each other's diagnoses and opinions in highly publicized court cases, leaving jurors and the public to doubt the validity of psychiatric testimony.[23] Many legal authorities refer to psychiatry as a "soft science" that lacks the objectivity, clarity, and reliability of the "hard sciences," such as forensic pathology. The soft science witness has been cynically and unfairly defined as "someone who was not there when it happened but for a fee will gladly imagine what it must have been like."[24] There is concern that psychiatric witnesses, at times, testify beyond their evidence, such as when they determine the mental status and responsibility of the defendant long after the crime has been committed. Finally, some judges have determined that many mental health and behavioral issues are within the scope of common knowledge and the average juror and do not require the expert opinion of a psychiatrist.[23]

The documentation of a mental injury presents a difficult challenge for the psychiatric witness. Many stress-related symptoms are essentially subjective and unverifiable. Because of the potential for distortion and symptom magnification for the sake of financial compensability, the accuracy of the patient's self-report must be carefully considered. At the same time, the possibility of underreporting psychiatric symptoms because of shame or embarrassment must also be taken into account. In performing one of the more perplexing tasks for a medical witness, the psychiatrist has to determine the legitimacy of the patient's subjective complaints and assess the possibility of malingering and exaggeration so that a fair settlement of the legal claim can be made.

In many cases, the psychiatrist will be asked about the patient's diagnosis as well as the patient's mental capacity to perform a certain task, such as the patient's ability to make a will or appreciate the wrongfulness of his or her conduct. The legally inexperienced psychiatrist may mistakenly equate any psychosis with a lack of legal capacity and responsibility. In fact, a schizophrenic with auditory hallucinations may still be knowledgeable about his or her own estate and be able to distinguish between right and wrong.

Psychiatric witnesses may encounter ethical dilemmas unique to their medical specialty. For example, a psychiatrist subpoenaed to court may provide confidential and sensitive information that could compromise the psychotherapist-client relationship or even harm the mental stability of the patient.[25] The psychiatrist will be in conflict between the duty to tell the whole truth to the court and the responsibility to prevent emotional harm to the patient. When the prospects of a psycholegal claim are apparent, the psychiatrist should inform the patient about the probability of the therapist being subpoenaed to testify, the potential loss of confidentiality, and the effects on the therapy relationship if the choice is made to proceed with a lawsuit. If the patient is agreeable to having the psychiatrist testify, it would be wise to obtain a signed consent form.

Another dilemma occurs when a psychiatrist is asked at a criminal trial to testify about the long-term dangerousness of defendants when the research evidence indicates that psychiatrists have no demonstrable expertise in such prognostications. The American Psychiatric Association has taken the position that the courts should disallow psychiatric testimony on long-term dangerousness, but the courts remain disinclined to prevent a psychiatrist from testifying as to future dangerousness and will continue to ask psychiatric witnesses to expound on that question.[26] Hence, psychiatrists who serve on sanity panels or testify at criminal trials should be prepared for a question like,

Q. Based on scientific knowledge, psychiatrists do not have the ability to predict future violent acts, isn't that true?

a. That's true. We can't make such predictions about future violence.

Psychiatric testimony in cases of dangerousness is not without some value for the jury. A more helpful reply is

A. Psychiatrists do not make such long-range predictions as that. But I can state with reasonable medical certainty that this woman, when she does not take her antipsychotic medication, has difficulty controlling her emotions and aggressive behavior.

Perhaps more so than other medical experts, psychiatrists will be challenged on the witness stand to substantiate their opinions with objective evidence and well-reasoned conclusions. In view of the bias generally held against psychiatry for being a soft science, it is imperative for the psychiatric witness to present intelligent and credible opinions because their testimony in civil and criminal court has important bearing on just settlements, family stability, and fundamental human rights.

Pathology and Radiology

Pathologists and radiologists provide essential medical support services in the clinical setting and have frequent entry into the medicolegal system. The reports of pathologists and radiologists are invariably included in civil and criminal cases and, because their data are among the most objective and concrete that medicine provides, the expertise of pathologists and radiologists are especially welcomed by the triers of fact.

Specialists in pathology, as a function of their duties in autopsy, are skilled in determining the time and cause of deaths. They are valuable in analyzing the effects of traumatic bodily injury, asphyxiation, gunshot wounds, burn injury, and chemical deaths, as well as alcohol and drug intoxication. The specialist in forensic pathology has, in addition to the work in the general field of pathology, a focused interest in legal cases that arise in civil and criminal courts, with responsibilities that range from disputed paternity suits to criminal investigations.

Pathologists enjoy the advantage of testifying on objective tests and hard evidence, and they do not have to contend with the subjective reports and exaggerated symptoms that other medical experts must endure.[2] Nonetheless, there are occasionally different opinions in pathology, such as estimating the time of death, which can place qualified and experienced pathologists at odds in the courtroom. Thus, even in a so-called hard science such as pathology, honest differences of opinion can be polarized into a "battle of experts," creating confusion and dismay among lay jurors who expect exact and indisputable scientific conclusions.[27]

In recent well-known criminal trials (e.g., the O.J. Simpson case and the Oklahoma City bombing trial), forensic experts have come under sharp criticism for the apparent mishandling of important trial evidence. The forensic pathologist is responsible for the preservation of medical evidence and has to account for its security to ensure that no altering or tampering has occurred. Although forensic pathologists must work closely with law enforcement officials and criminal attorneys in preparing for trials, they should maintain an independent position in all matters and testify as impartial scientific witnesses.

Beeman[28] described several different types of medical witnesses among pathologists. There is the dogmatist who, as a result of hindsight in examining tissues and fluids, is self-anointed with infallibility. The academician is the pathologist who is a knowledgeable scientist and can be a valuable witness if adaptable to the ambience of the courtroom. Beeman found the average pathologist to be competent and honest but uncomfortable with lawyers and court proceedings. He concluded that the ideal witness is one who is competent and experienced, sensitive to the limits of his or her expertise, and well aware of trial procedures and legal strategies.

The work of specialists in radiology is ubiquitous in one form or another at legal hearings. As a matter of law, many jurisdictions have held that, if testimony based on diagnostic imaging is admitted into evidence, the x-ray films or CT and MRI scans must be shown in court and often become official exhibits.[29]

The radiologist witness must be adept at explaining the results of x-ray studies and scans to laypeople. If the diagnostic test is not one of the more routine procedures known to the average person, the radiologist has to describe the procedure itself. Like the pathologist witness, the radiology expert is responsible for the management of the medical evidence to be used at hearings and therefore must preserve its security and be able to identify with certainty the test results of the particular patient.

At times the terminology used to describe radiology results can be misunderstood by lay jurors. Consequently, the radiologist must be able to clarify commonly used medical terms such as "bulging," "protruding," or "herniated," because these findings are not readily visualized by the untrained eye. The explanation of technical jargon into everyday language is a vital role of the radiologist witness to project the solid findings that diagnostic imaging offers.

With regard to malpractice lawsuits against radiologists, the claims of missed diagnosis represent nearly one-half of the cases. In the past, fractures were the most common undetected abnormalities, but recently the failure to detect lung cancer on x-ray films has become the most frequent complaint of the failure to diagnose.[30] Although the medicolegal charge is usually on a missed diagnosis, the false-positive reading is equally important because it may lead to subsequent diagnostic tests that may be hazardous to the patient.[31] The potential sources of negligent events in radiology are several, including image quality, lesion detection, lesion recognition, and communication of the results to the referring physician. The best protection against malpractice complaints for the radiologist is the consistent maintenance of proper standards of care, including knowledge of the sensitivity and specificity of radiography for the detection of cancers as well as the indications for additional diagnostic procedures.

Closing Arguments

The interface between the law and medical specialists is manifold, and each specialty has its unique medicolegal responsibilities and courtroom challenges. The specialists discussed in this chapter will probably be involved in more legal activity than their other colleagues, but in this era of low thresholds for litigation, all physicians should be prepared to receive at one time or another in their professional career a subpoena to testify at a hearing for one of their patients. The admonishments for all specialists remain the same: practice high standards of medicine, maintain good patient records, know the strengths and limits of your expertise, learn about the legal system as it pertains to your medical specialty, and be an impartial witness who advocates not for a patient or attorney but for the truth.

References

1. Horsley JE. *Testifying in Court: A Guide for Physicians* (4th ed). Los Angeles: Product Management Information Corp., 1992.
2. Curran WJ. *Tracy's The Doctor as a Witness* (2nd ed). Philadelphia: Saunders, 1965.
3. Beresford HR. *Legal Aspects of Neurologic Practice: Contemporary Neurology Series.* Philadelphia: FA Davis, 1975.
4. Ennis M, Clark A, Grudzinskas JG. Change in obstetric practice in response to fear of litigation in the British Isles. *Lancet* 1991;338:616–618.
5. Symonds EM. Obstetrics and Gynaecology. In JP Jackson (ed), *A Practical Guide to Medicine and the Law.* London: Springer-Verlag, 1991;45–75.
6. Boenning DA, Selbst SM, Freed LH, Groves AM. The pediatrician as expert witness: participation and reaction to this activity. *Pediatr Legal Med* 1992;146:1107–1109.
7. Strodel RC. *Securing and Using Medical Evidence in Personal Injury and Health-Care Cases.* Englewood, NJ: Prentice-Hall, 1988.
8. Danner D, Sagall EL. Medicolegal causation: a source of professional misunderstanding. *Am J Law Med* 1977;3:303–308.

9. Leaman TL, Saxton JW. *Preventing Malpractice: The Co-Active Solution.* New York: Plenum Medical, 1993.
10. Hahn RG, Lefever RD, Geagan J. The family physician as a legal consultant. *J Family Pract* 1985;20:569–572.
11. Keddie, N. General Surgery. In JP Jackson (ed), *A Practical Guide to Medicine and the Law.* London: Springer-Verlag, 1991;77–94.
12. Shandell RE. *The Preparation and Trial of Medical Malpractice Cases.* New York: Law Journal Seminars Press, 1981.
13. American Medical Association. *Guides to the Evaluation of Permanent Impairment* (4th ed). Washington, DC: American Medical Association, 1993.
14. Goodman HF. *Orthopedic Disability and Expert Testimony* (4th ed). New York: Wiley Law, 1993.
15. Quality Standards Subcommittee of the American Academy of Neurology. Practice parameters for determining brain death in adults (summary statement). *Neurology* 1995;45:1012–1014.
16. Glosser DS. Medicolegal considerations in postconcussive syndrome. In WH Simon, GE Ehrlich (eds), *Medicolegal Consequences of Trauma.* New York: Marcel Dekker, 1993;473–495.
17. Godwin-Austen RB. Neurology. In JP Jackson (ed), *A Practical Guide to Medicine and the Law.* London: Springer-Verlag, 1991;137–155.
18. Rosenberg NL. Neurotoxicity. In JB Sullivan, GR Krieger (eds), *Hazardous Materials Toxicology.* Baltimore: Williams & Wilkins, 1992; 145–153.
19. Robertson JD, Keavy WT. *Plastic Surgery Malpractice and Damages.* Somerset, NJ: Wiley, 1990.
20. Angell M. Do breast implants cause systemic disease? Science in the courtroom. *N Engl J Med* 1994;330:1748–1749.
21. Rosenberg NL. The neuromythology of silicone breast implants. *Neurology* 1996;46:308–314.
22. Blinder M. *Psychiatry in the Everyday Practice of Law* (3rd ed). Deerfield, IL: Clark Boardman Callaghan, 1992.
23. Chaplow DG, Peters JL, Kydd RR. The expert witness in forensic psychiatry. *Aust N Z J Psychiatry* 1992;26:624–630.
24. Tigar ME. *Examining Witnesses.* Chicago: American Bar Association, 1993.
25. Appelbaum PS, Gutheil TG. *Clinical Handbook of Psychiatry and the Law* (3rd ed). Baltimore: Williams & Wilkins, 1991.
26. Goldsmith MF. Psychiatric testimony: what are its limits? *JAMA* 1984; 252:186–187, 191.
27. Craighead JE. The pathologist as an expert witness. *Arch Pathol Lab Med* 1992;116: 488–489.
28. Beeman J. *The Pathologist as a Witness.* Mundelein, IL: Callaghan, 1964.
29. Berlin L, Berlin JW. Malpractice and radiologists in Cook County, IL: trends in 20 years of litigation. *AJR Am J Roentgenol* 1995;165:781–788.
30. Hamer M, Morlock F, Foley HT, Ros PR. Medical malpractice in diagnostic radiology: claims, compensation, and patient injury. *Radiology* 1987;164:263–266.
31. Potchen EJ, Bisesi MA. When is it malpractice to miss lung cancer on chest radiographs? *Radiology* 1990;175:29–32.

9

The Deposition

Since about 1946, federal and state laws have evolved asserting that the interests of justice are best served by allowing opposing parties in a lawsuit access to relevant evidence in each other's possession or control. Theoretically, such access provides the attorneys with thorough discovery techniques and preparation of cases, eliminates the element of surprise at future trials, promotes justice, and may encourage out-of-court settlements by offering the opposing attorneys the opportunity to assess the strengths and weaknesses of their cases.

Discovery techniques are those procedures by which supporting evidence becomes disclosed, and they include interrogatories, depositions, and various subpoenas for the production of documents. Discovery may be invoked by any party to the lawsuit, and the court in which the suit is filed administers the discovery proceedings.

The rules governing discovery procedures differ from one jurisdiction to another, although most states have adopted entirely, or with slight modifications, the Federal Civil Judicial Procedures and Rules.[1] Generally, courts rather freely grant motions for discovery provided that there exists some indication that the data to be discovered are indeed relevant. Discovery is intended to be as extensive as possible in order to avoid a "trial by ambush." However, courts do not kindly regard blanket requests by attorneys for evidence of doubtful relevance, that is, the so-called fishing expedition.

During the discovery phase, both sides of the lawsuit identify individuals who will be witnesses at the trial. These witnesses are then available for examination by the opposing lawyer before trial in order to determine what their testimony will be. The physician's entry into the legal process will occur during this phase of discovery. The physician will be provided with written questions, known as *interrogatories,* to elicit the physician's knowledge of the case. Most attorneys, however, will proceed to request from the physician a face-to-face oral examination, known as a *deposition,* in which they are permitted to pose questions that the medical witness is required to answer as though on the witness stand in open court.

A deposition is the most commonly used legal process employed in the discovery phase and is designed to obtain a sworn testimony from a key witness or party to the lawsuit. Applicable laws pertaining to the nature and extent of discovery obtained through oral depositions depend on the Rules of Civil Procedures, rules of the circuit court, statutes of evidence, and case law of individual states and jurisdictions. The potential physician witness must become familiar with these laws that govern the obtaining of evidence, or at least confer with an attorney regarding issues such as confidential medical records.

Attorneys for either party may seek a deposition by obtaining an order from the appropriate court directing the witness, or deponent, to appear at a designated time and place for purposes of questioning about matters relevant to issues in the suit. When a physician receives a subpoena to attend a deposition, arrangements should be made to meet with "your" attorney. (If the physician is to testify as a treating doctor, the deposition is usually being requested by an opposing attorney who represents the defendant and, for the sake of this chapter, "your attorney" refers to the lawyer retained by your patient. If the physician is to testify as a nontreating consultant, then "your attorney" is the lawyer who has retained you for your expert opinions.) Your attorney can explain to you the pertinent medicolegal matters, including the nature of the legal claim, the information produced thus far by discovery, and the central medical issues that are likely to arise during the deposition. In turn, you can inform your attorney about the nature of the medical evidence you possess, explaining the strengths and weaknesses in the data you are going to present.

In many states there is a "medical-legal interprofessional courtesy agreement" accepted by the local medical and legal boards and authorities. The courtesy agreement consists of general policies that guide both professions regarding cooperation with depositions and fee schedules. You are advised to clearly discuss with your attorney matters of expert fees, costs of reviewing records, giving the deposition, and other related costs.

Preparing for Depositions

In preparing for the deposition, request from your attorney a full set of records pertaining to the case. You may have to direct the attorney to obtain certain documents that have not yet been obtained—for example, computed tomographic (CT) scans and technical studies, work history, or prior criminal records. In some cases you should obtain information of your own, such as a more current examination of the patient and interviews with family members or employers. Inquire as to the other medical experts involved in the case. Obtain their reports and documents, such as test results. Review their resumes if possible to fully assess their potential contributions to the case. If you do not obtain these relevant data before the deposition, you can do so afterward, but if the additional information will alter your testimony at trial in any way, the opposing attorney has the right to order another deposition from you. As stated earlier, the aim of the discovery process is to avoid any unexpected testimony in the courtroom.

Your attorney can be a valuable source of possible questions that the deposing lawyer may ask, as well as information about the opposing counsel's style of questioning and usual strategies. Through your discussions with your attorney you can learn how to best present your evidence. However, your attorney cannot and should not provide answers for you. You are legally and ethically bound to offer *your* own professional opinions, not those of your patient or your attorney. Make clear to your attorney the limits of your evidence as well as your level of expertise. Some lawyers may want more from you than is warranted by your data or your competency.

You should work closely with your attorney, but you must resist forming an alliance with counsel. To maintain your impartiality and objectivity, you cannot join in the advocacy for the attorney's side of the case. Physicians are advocates for the patient in the doctor-patient relationship, but in a court of law, you must advocate for the *truth* and not the patient.

Preparing well-worded responses to difficult questions is a good idea, but rehearsing or memorizing answers is not recommended because it can result in giving the appearance of overly prepared, canned answers or, worse, in possible mental blocking during the deposition that will result in blanks and major gaps in your testimony. A natural conversational flow is more impressive and convincing. Finally, whatever is discussed with your attorney before the deposition can be queried by the opposing lawyer at the time of the deposition and put on record.

The subpoena that orders you to appear for the deposition will introduce you to the attorney or attorneys on the opposing side. Before the deposition, you may receive a telephone call from the deposing attorney clarifying the time and place of the deposition as well as your fees for testifying. If you have contact with the opposing lawyer, you should be careful not to make any informal statements about the case, because your remarks can be brought up in the deposition or trial. If asked about the case, tell the attorney that you prefer to answer the questions at the deposition.

Just before the deposition, review your clinical records and notes on the patient. You want to have at your fingertips exact dates, clinical findings, and conclusions. You need not commit these specific facts to memory because you are permitted to consult your records during the deposition. Be very clear about the reasoning process underlying your evidence and conclusion. Be aware of the limits of your knowledge on the case and be prepared to say "I don't know" when appropriate.

Be familiar with the law and legal terms relevant to your testimony. For example, you will be asked to offer opinions based on *reasonable medical certainty*. Reasonable medical certainty does not mean absolute certainty or the highest level of scientific probability. As indicated in Chapter 1, in civil law, reasonable medical certainty means "more likely than not" or "preponderance (51%) of the evidence." Applying the strictest medical standards in civil cases would be incorrect and unjust.[2]

Purposes and Goals of Depositions

The most basic goal of the deposition is to prepare for trial by discovering what facts and arguments will be presented in the courtroom. A deposition gives the opposing side a fair chance to prepare rebuttals to all contentions being made in the case. With a physician witness, the opposing attorney will ask many detailed questions in an effort to know what medical evidence will be presented and the reasoning behind the opinions rendered. In addition to this basic aim, there can be several other purposes for the deposition of an expert witness.[3,4]

The deposing attorney wants to obtain a sworn testimony from the witness to commit the witness to certain statements and preserve the testimony, which can be used as evidence later at trial (e.g., as impeachment evidence if the deponent alters an opinion in court). In the deposition, the opposing counsel can confront the expert witness with conflicting evidence or opinions and observe the deponent's ability to explain the weaknesses in the case. The deposition presents an opportunity to assess the physician's skill and demeanor as a witness. In addition to inquiring about the physician's professional credentials, the opposing counsel wants to see how persuasive the physician is, how the expert copes with the rigors of cross-examination, and what kind of impression will be made with the jurors.

The Physician Witness's Role in Depositions

At a deposition, the role of the opposing attorney, as the advocate for the other side, is to search for information that will help his or her client's case. What, then, is the role of the physician deponent? According to Federal Rules of Evidence 702, the expert witness's raison d'etre is to assist the triers of fact in understanding the evidence or a fact in evidence. Legal authorities generally agree that the basic function of the deposition witness is to listen carefully to each question and answer responsively and accurately.

However, there are no set guidelines for the role of an expert witness in a deposition. Some, such as Appelbaum and Gutheil,[5] assert that the expert witness in offering opinions should neither overstate the certainty of the conclusions reached nor understate the possibility of alternative viewpoints. Benjamin and Kaszniak[3] indicate that an expert witness should report the results of the available evidence and function as an educator, not an advocate. In contrast, Zobel and Rous[4] postulate that the expert has no duty to provide educational services and explicitly state, "A deposition is not Grand Rounds."

According to certain legal experts,[4,6,7] the expert witness's approach in a deposition is an entirely different exercise than testifying in a courtroom. At a trial, the physician witness in direct examination may assume the role of a teacher and be somewhat expansive in answering questions. At a deposition, which is a discovery procedure for the opposing counsel in search of how to discredit the expert's testimony, the deponent is advised to be relatively brief and to the point. Thus, the physician witness is advised to respond succinctly to questions and not provide answers that the deposing attorney has not asked for specifically, following the adage, "Never volunteer unsolicited information."

Because the deposing attorney is highly interested in obtaining information with which to discredit the witness, Rossi[6] further admonishes the deponent "to keep his guard up at all times" and advises expert witnesses to "make them beat answers out of you." If more information is desired from the deponent, it is the opposing counsel's responsibility to follow up with additional questions, which the witness should answer responsively.

The advice from legal authorities varies, but they agree that the deponent is obligated to answer each question as truthfully and accurately as possible, regardless of which side has retained the witness.

The Deposition

The deposition is usually conducted during business hours in the offices of the deposing attorney or often at the office of the physician witness out of courtesy and because of the availability of the medical documents. At the deposition, those present include the physician witness or deponent, the attorneys from both sides, and a court reporter who is also a notary public to administer the oath. The patient is usually not present.

Sometimes the opposing attorney will employ a medical consultant who will be present in order to suggest lines of questioning based on the discovery documents or the witness's answers at the deposition. The opposing expert can also assess the qualifications and capabilities of the deponent.

Under the rules in most jurisdictions, the deposition can proceed in any manner and to whatever extent the two opposing attorneys agree upon. The rules do not limit the length of the deposition or the number of depositions. The deponent can bring materials that may assist, such as notes and reference books, although one should be prepared for questions that could be asked about the notes or textbooks.

After the deponent is sworn in, the deposing attorney will begin by explaining the basic ground rules that govern depositions. One of the first requests is to ask the deponent to provide a current resume or curriculum vitae (CV). Have your CV available with a precise listing of your educational background, licenses and board certifications, professional experiences, medical societies, and any awards or honors you have received. Some physicians have developed a CV used for public relations and promotional purposes, with a generous embellishing of credentials and skills. These kinds of resumes raise concerns about a physician's tendency to exaggerate and be self-serving and should not be submitted to the other side.

It is easy for a physician witness to misunderstand the significance of a deposition.[7] Because the proceedings are held in the comfort of their offices, physicians sometimes forget that they are speaking under oath and are subject to all the rules, responsibilities, and penalties of testifying in a courtroom. In the daily routines of medical practice in their offices, a physician forms many opinions, including solid medical judgments as well as speculations and "gut feelings," such as, "Yes, the lung cancer could be due to his exposure to asbestos at work." During a deposition, the physician must limit opinions to those based on reasonable medical certainty and should avoid speculations and guesses. If you casually offer a guess (e.g., "I guess the therapy worsened her condition"), you cannot later give a more precise testimony at trial (e.g., "I'm certain the therapy worsened her condition").

It should be noted that certain attorneys have a casual and friendly approach, enticing the witness to let down his or her guard, engage in a free-flowing conversation, and provide more detailed responses than are necessary. Depositions appear relatively informal, but any statement made can be introduced as evidence during the actual trial, and the deposition testimony cannot be changed. Moreover, knowingly making a false statement in a deposition constitutes perjury. Keep in mind that what is said at a deposition becomes a permanent record that can be used again months or even years afterwards.

Tips for the Physician Deponent

In a deposition, as in court, a physician witness should listen carefully and patiently to each question. You should listen to *all* the words in a question before answering. Physicians who dislike being deposed and resent the time spent on nonmedical business overly anticipate questions, answer prematurely, and even volunteer answers to questions not yet asked. A question you consider harmless and want to quickly answer may be potentially damaging. If you blurt out an answer before your attorney can warn you with an objection, the damage is done. The skilled medical expert will resist these temptations and will consider questions carefully before speaking.

Take your time to answer questions; your pauses will not be reflected in the deposition transcript. A brief pause after the question is asked gives your attorney a better chance to form appropriate objections, and it gives you time to think of a good answer. Objections are made by your attorney for legal reasons (e.g., vague and ambiguous question, question already asked and answered, lack of foundation, question wrongly assumes expertise the witness does not have) or for strategic purposes, such as assisting the witness by interrupting a series of stressful questions and giving the deponent time to think of a good answer. Generally these objections are for the record to be determined later by a judge, and you still have to respond to the question. Follow your attorney's direction; if you are told not to answer, stop talking. If the other lawyer says, "Go ahead and answer," do not automatically answer the question. Your attorney may state "You may answer the question" or give you a look of approval, at which point you can resume talking.

Whenever you answer, speak slowly, clearly, and loudly enough so that the court reporter can accurately record your response. Speak in complete sentences, as if you are dictating an important report. Avoid nonverbal communication, such as head-shaking or nodding, which cannot be recorded. Similarly, responses such as "uh-huh" or "uh-uh" are ambiguous and create problems for the court reporter. Describe any letter or document that you comment on in the deposition (e.g., "This is my letter to the patient dated . . ." or "On this sheet entitled 'Emergency Room Report' . . .").

Ambiguous Questions

If the deposing attorney asks an ambiguous question, do not try to answer it. For example,

Q. Doctor, was the patient better before the accident?

Instead of assuming what is meant by "better" or "before," you should ask for the question to be restated or rephrased. You can ask for more specifics or additional background. Consider these responses:

A. What do you mean by "better"?

A. I don't understand. Can you restate the question?

A. I'm sorry. Please rephrase the question.

A. How long before the accident are you referring to?

A. Can you be more specific?

Paraphrasing

You are advised not to paraphrase an ambiguous question. Your version of the question may suggest different ideas not considered by the opposing counsel, and you may be offering unsolicited information. For instance,

    a. Are you asking, "Was she better *emotionally* before the accident?"

    a. Do you want to know about her *general health* or about her *work performance*?

    a. If you mean, "Was she in better health?," the answer is "Yes." If you mean, "Was she a better person?," the answer is "No." The accident has made her re-evaluate her priorities and she's a better person now.

These three responses might offer new ideas to the cross-examiner and provide information not necessarily requested in the question.

Taking Breaks

If at any time you want to take a break or consult with your attorney, a recess can be taken. A brief time-out is helpful during a grueling deposition. The break can help you regain composure. However, do not overuse this privilege. Frequent consultations with your attorney will make you appear incompetent, fearful, or manipulative. Moreover, the deposing attorney could state for the record,

    Q. Doctor, you've had your third recess to consult with your attorney. Are you ready to continue with this deposition?

Just as at the courthouse, refrain from talking to anyone at the deposition except your counsel. Comments made during a break in the hallway, in the bathroom, or "off the record" can be used by the deposing attorney to put on the record. Making social conversation, you may casually say, "This was a difficult patient to care for" or "I'm not surprised this case has ended up in a lawsuit." Comments like these can be brought into the deposition and further explored by the opposing attorney.

Q. Doctor, why did you say during the break that you're not surprised this case has ended up in a lawsuit?

Lawyers at a deposition often engage in friendly banter, ranging from teasing and joking to sarcasms and overstatements. With a barroom atmosphere, it may be tempting to join in the repartee with off-color remarks such as "He wasn't a crock like some of my other patients" or "Well, maybe she had PMS." Everything said is being recorded and when read in court the physician can only be seen as crude, insensitive, and unprofessional. The lawyers can afford to bring some wit into the proceedings; physician witnesses should remain professional in all of their responses at a deposition.

Double Negatives

Listen very carefully to double or triple negative questions, such as

Q. Wouldn't you say that were it not for the accident the patient would be without injuries?

With questions containing multiple negatives, answer with care so as not to leave the wrong impression. For example,

Q. You don't have an opinion about future medical costs, do you?

If you don't have an opinion you might incorrectly say "No" when the correct answer is "Yes." To be certain that you are not misunderstood, do not answer with a simple "Yes" or "No." Instead say,

A. Yes. I don't have an opinion about future medical costs.

or,

A. No. I do have an opinion about future medical costs.

Compound Questions

Be aware of compound questions, especially if part of the question is not accurate. For example,

Q. After you briefly looked at the patient's injuries, what conclusions did you reach?

a. I concluded that her injuries were not serious.

This answer implies an agreement that the physician *quickly* looked at the patient's injuries. A more careful response would be

A. I looked at the patient's injuries carefully, not briefly, and I concluded that her injuries were not serious.

Nonsystematic Questioning

The questioning in a deposition may go in any direction the lawyer wishes. The sequence of questions may not be logical or chronological and may shift quickly from topic to topic. Deposing attorneys may do this to keep the witness off balance and not in control of the flow of the discussion.

Jumping from one subject to another may frustrate the deponent because it may prevent the witness from completing the entire thought on the subject matter. Control your need to set the record straight, because your additional comments may simply result in your giving the opposing counsel more material to attack.

Differing with Other Physicians

When your medical opinion differs from that of other physicians, you can expect to be challenged in the following way:

Q. Doctor, isn't it true that your conclusions contradict that of the two other doctors testifying in this trial?

A. Yes.

Q. Why is that?

A. I don't know.

Q. In the past, have you differed in your opinions with other doctors?

a. Yes.

Q. Has this happened often?

a. Yes.

The last two "Yes" answers, without further elaboration, can lead the jurors to believe that the witness's opinion is often different, unusual, or possibly wrong. Physicians often disagree on medical matters, and the witness should explain:

A. Doctors do not always agree in their diagnoses and opinions. I don't know about the other two doctors in this case, but I am certain that my diagnosis is based on objective findings and a thorough evaluation of the patient.

Changing Your Testimony

You should be aware that attorneys sometimes rephrase your testimony with subtle changes that favor their side of the case. For example,

Q. Doctor, you have told us that the plaintiff fell and struck his head, isn't that true?

A. Yes.

Q. And your testimony is that he has suffered head trauma and brain damage, correct?

A. No. I said he has suffered a head trauma and shows evidence of brain dysfunction because of his memory impairment. At this point, I do not know if he has actual brain damage.

The message once again is: Pay close attention to each question. Every word counts. Do not agree with any restatement unless it accurately reflects your testimony.

Analyzing Questions

Do not try to analyze the reasons behind the lawyer's questions. Just answer the question. For instance,

Q. Do you trust what the patient tells you?

a. Now, don't think I only relied on what the patient said. I thoroughly reviewed his medical records and even called his previous physician.

Your defensiveness and argumentativeness will show that you can be easily rattled in court. The above question deserves a simple answer.

A. Yes.

Open-Ended Questions

Be cautious about answering broad open-ended questions intended to elicit information that could be used to discredit your testimony.

Q. What are the causes of thoracic outlet syndrome?

Q. How is a thorough examination done for this kind of disorder?

Q. What are some of the ways you can treat this illness?

Q. Tell us, what are some of the ways doctors make erroneous diagnoses?

You have a duty to answer these questions directly and accurately, but you are not required to elaborate at length or give information not essential to the question being asked.[6] Some physicians, perhaps with a personal need to prove their competency, will provide a short lecture instead of a terse but adequate response. If you choose to be verbose, be prepared to answer many follow-up questions that may emerge from your speech.

Your Attorney's Questions

After the deposing attorney has completed the questioning, your attorney will have an opportunity to ask questions and will do so primarily to clarify some of your opinions or to rectify any misleading statements you may have made. Because the deposition is a discovery process for the opposing side, your attorney will ask very few questions so as to avoid volunteering any information not requested by the deposing lawyer. Your attorney will question you at length if you will not be available for the trial, with your deposition to be used as evidence at the trial. (The most frequent reason for expert witnesses being excused from testifying in court is if they live more than 100 miles from the courthouse.[2])

Locking Up Your Testimony

Toward the end of the deposition, the opposing attorney will attempt to place constraints on any future opinions or modifications by the physician witness by asking,

Q. Are those the only problems the patient has?

Q. Do you have any other opinion that you have not expressed on this case?

Q. Have we covered all areas that you will testify about on this case?

These questions are efforts to lock up the testimony so that the expert witness cannot add comments or changes at trial. The deponent is advised not to answer these questions with a simple "Yes" but to leave an opening for later modifications or additions to your testimony.

A. Based on the facts available, these are the only problems I can recall at this time.

A. As far as I know now I don't have anything else to say.

A. I believe we have covered the major areas at this time. I will continue to study this case and would be glad to tell you of any opinions on this case that may come up in the future.

Reviewing the Deposition Transcript

When the deposition questioning ends, the court reporter will ask, "Doctor, will you waive the signature?" The court reporter is asking you if you want to read a copy of the deposition transcript and sign it. It is important for you not to waive your right to proofread your deposition statements for incorrect spelling of names, diagnoses, tests, and medications and also to find errors or omissions, such as an important "not" which can wrongly represent your testimony. Thus, do not answer "Yes" to the court reporter. Insist on receiving a copy of the deposition transcript and carefully proofread it.

The deposition transcript is not routinely admissible as evidence in any trial that follows. However, it will be used as evidence if statements in the deposition contradict the deponent's subsequent testimony at trial. Thus, it behooves you to protect yourself against any inaccurate representation of your opinions. Otherwise, the deposition testimony may not only become an embarrassment but, worse, a basis for impeachment at trial. Under the federal rules, the deponent has 30 days to make changes after receipt of the transcript. Otherwise the reporter will file the uncorrected and unsigned transcript as an enduring record of your opinion. Usually you are given a copy of the deposition for your records so that you can review it in preparing for the trial.

If the deposition elicits clear, well-supported responses from a competent expert witness that weigh substantially against his or her client, the deposing attorney may seek to resolve the lawsuit without risking a loss in court. Conversely, if the deponent provides weak evidence or becomes easily shaken, the attorney may relish the chance to undermine the expert witness's testimony on cross-examination at a subsequent trial. Even if the prospects of settlement of the case are not affected, a deposition may be quite helpful to attorneys on both sides in preparing for trial since they will know in advance the essential testimony of the deponent.

Video Deposition

When an expert witness is not available for a trial, the use of a videotaped deposition may be obtained for trial. Several unique challenges arise in providing a video deposition that are not problems when giving a stenographic oral deposition. Whereas the jury listening to a third-party reading of the physician witness's conventional oral deposition digest only words, with a video deposition the jurors see everything. The jurors closely observe how the medical witness sounds and looks during the testimony.

The jury will carefully pay attention to the physical appearance of the deponent. Jurors anticipate that the physician witness will match their sartorial expectations. Generally, attire should be sufficiently conventional to blend into the background unobserved. What you wear should not distract from what you say. Flashy jewelry, gaudy accessories, pagers, and other distracting items should not be in the camera's view. Preferably you should schedule a taping in the morning to present a fresh appearance in clothing and hygiene (e.g., avoid the 5 o'clock shadow).

The medical expert witness deposed on videotape must be careful not to exhibit nonverbal behavior that might be perceived as a negative or uncooperative attitude. Hesitant delivery, avoidance of eye contact with counsel, slouching, smirking, appearing impatient or disgusted with questions, wringing of hands, and other gestures that are concealed in written depositions become glaringly significant when televised to the jury. The goal is to appear confident and be responsive and candid while nevertheless scrupulously observing the same cautions one would in a stenographic oral deposition. You should be forthright and cooperative while carefully providing only that information which is specifically requested by the deposing counsel.

Video recordings can be unforgiving to physician witnesses playing strictly by the rules of the legal system. Limiting answers to terse "yes" or "no" responses or asking the deposing lawyer to further clarify a question that the jury already understands may be an effective strategy in conventional oral depositions, but it may alienate jurors viewing the same approach on video. As experienced television viewers, the jury might consider such tactics evasive or suspiciously combative. Resorting to sarcasms, caustic humor, or arguing with attorneys will also portray a negative image to those watching the video.

Video cameras dramatically exacerbate an expert witness's sense of anxiety. Remember that stage fright is natural. Rather than trying to suppress it, you should learn to channel the anxiety into positive energy and a spirited testimony. To relieve excessive tension, you can employ deep breathing, neck and shoulder rolls, and calming imagery techniques before the video deposition. A calm witness will project greater confidence and credibility, which are essential for effective testifying.

Expressing emotions relevant to the testimony shows the jury that the medical witness is as human as they are. Expressed appropriately, lively emotive communications help to persuade the jury that you are convinced of your conclusions and will promote credibility and empathy. Combativeness and anger will be a disadvantage, whereas enthusiasm, certainty, and even justified indignation at outrageous questions will be beneficial for the testifying witness.

Frequently during a video recording you need to remind yourself to slow down and reflect for a moment before answering. The anxiety engendered by the camera causes witnesses to forget the practice of taking a momentary pause. Instead, the witness often feels pressure that can lead to inarticulate and damaging answers.

An effective communicative tool in videotaping will be demonstrative aids, such as charts that allow you to explain the case visually. When using exhibits or other visual aids, you should continue to turn toward the camera and maintain eye contact.

Repeated on-camera role-playing of the deposition will improve the communication abilities of the physician witness. An effective video deposition, like other presentations on imaging media (e.g., television), consists of a good performance.

Closing Arguments

Physicians are more likely to undergo an oral deposition in their offices than to testify in court, but they continue to misunderstand this vital phase of a legal case. Because of the relatively informal atmosphere of being questioned away from the courtroom and in the comfort of one's own offices, it is easy to forget that a deposition is, like testifying on the witness stand, a sworn testimony with the same rules and penalties connected with a real trial. Every opinion provided is a final opinion, that is, you cannot change your statements at a subsequent trial without risking impeachment of your entire testimony. Thus, it is essential to prepare thoroughly for the deposition by reviewing the medical records as well as your own reports and meeting with your attorney to discuss the medical and legal aspects of the case. Without preparation and forethought, you will likely offer poorly considered statements that you cannot retract later.

The deposition differs in important ways from the courtroom testimony. The deposition is a discovery mechanism for the opposing attorney who wants to learn not only your findings and opinions but also the weaknesses in your position and how you react to and handle difficult questions. All of this is valuable to the opposing counsel in preparing to cross-examine you at trial.

This chapter revealed some of the goals and strategies of a deposing attorney. Knowing what the opposing lawyer is after will ease some of your apprehensions and prepare you to handle the deposition more effectively. Do not let this knowledge tempt you into engaging in tactical one-upmanship with the opposing counsel. You can be cautious about open-ended questions but you should not resist questions or be uncooperative. Most of all, do not try to outwit the lawyer. This is a legal proceeding and you are no match for experienced attorneys working on their own turf.

A deposition is often a negative experience for the medical witness. The questioning is primarily one-sided. The deposing lawyer has noted some limitations in your training or professional experience. Flaws in your data-gathering have been revealed. Opposing arguments seem persuasive. Do not be discombobulated by these occurrences. The very purpose of a deposition is to search for weaknesses in your statements and to discredit and possibly impeach your testimony; the opposing lawyer did not depose you to applaud your expertise.

Your best insurance for a successful deposition is to be prepared to support your opinions with solid scientific evidence and cogent medical reasoning, not speculation or unsupported assumptions. You will help yourself most by providing a clear, succinct, accurate, and intelligible presentation of your findings, and you may in the process also help the attorneys on both sides reach a satisfactory out-of-court settlement of the legal dispute.

References

1. *Federal Civil Judicial Procedures and Rules*. St. Paul, MN: West, 1991.
2. Liebenson HA. *You, the Expert Witness*. Mundelein, IL: Callaghan, 1962.
3. Benjamin GAH, Kaszniak A. The Discovery Process: Deposition, Trial Testimony, and Hearing Testimony. In HO Doerr, AS Carlin (eds), *Forensic Neuropsychology: Legal and Scientific Bases*. New York: Guilford Press, 1991;17–32.
4. Zobel HB, Rous SN. *Doctors and the Law*. New York: WW Norton, 1993.
5. Appelbaum PS, Gutheil TG. *Clinical Handbook of Psychiatry and the Law* (2nd ed). Baltimore: Williams & Wilkins, 1991.
6. Rossi FF. *Expert Witnesses*. Chicago: American Bar Association, 1991.
7. Horsley JE. *Testifying in Court: A Guide for Physicians* (4th ed). Los Angeles: Product Information Management, 1992.

10

Sample Deposition

This chapter consists of a sample oral deposition taken from a neurologist who treated a person injured in a traffic accident. To incorporate as many different challenges as possible, the questions and responses are excerpts taken from the actual depositions of several different cases blended into a single deposition.

The case involves a 32-year-old man who was the driver of a car that was rear-ended by another car, causing a minor closed-head injury along with neck and back injuries. The patient underwent standard conservative treatment including anti-inflammatory medication, mild analgesics, and physical therapy. Because of complaints of memory impairment and persistent headaches, the patient was also administered a battery of neuropsychological tests and received a series of biofeedback therapy. A complicating factor in this medicolegal case was the pre-existing back condition from an earlier work-related injury.

Examination

Q. Doctor, please state your full name for the record.

A. I'm Dr. Robert Anderson.

Q. What is your business address?

A. My office is at Straub Clinic, 888 South King Street, Honolulu, Hawaii, 96813.

Q. Doctor, I am Mr. Vincent and I represent the defendant in this case. Ms. Stevens, who is also present, is the attorney for the plaintiff and your patient, Mr. Green.

A. I see.

Q. Now, Doctor, your deposition is being taken today because the records show that you're one of the physicians who have treated Mr. Green. Is that correct?

A. Yes.

Attorney Gives Deposition Instructions

Q. Doctor, I take it that you've had a deposition taken before.

A. That's right.

Q. You understand that this is a legal proceeding in which your sworn testimony is being taken as if you're testifying in a court of law.

A. Yes.

Q. Everything you say will be reproduced in a transcript form. You'll have an opportunity to review that transcript, Doctor, but you understand that if you make changes to that transcript, I can comment about it to the jury and judge. So, in order for that not to happen, you are required to testify to the best of your ability and your knowledge in this case. Is that understood, Doctor?

A. Yes.

Q. One more thing. Plaintiff counsel may make an objection to my questions. This is because the objections must be made now, to preserve them for the record. You will be expected to answer the question anyway. Okay?

A. That's fine.

Attorney Inquires about Witness's Qualifications

Q. Doctor, we have your curriculum vitae here and I'm going to ask that it be marked as Exhibit 1 and attached. I'm not going to ask you about everything that's in the CV, but I'm going to go through some of the main points. First of all, are you a medical doctor?

A. Yes.

Q. And in what states are you licensed?

A. Massachusetts, California, and Hawaii.

Q. Is your primary practice here in Hawaii?

A. Yes.

Q. And you're affiliated with a particular group or facility?

A. Yes. I'm with Straub Clinic and Hospital, Inc., in Honolulu.

Q. How long have you been with Straub Clinic?

A. Twenty-one years.

Q. Doctor, please give us a brief summary of your educational background and medical training.

A. Okay. I received a Bachelor of Arts degree from Pomona College in Claremont, California. I received a medical degree from Columbia University in New York City. I also received a Master of Public Health degree from Harvard University and a Master of Science degree in Epidemiology from Harvard. I did my internship at Queen's Medical Center in Honolulu, and I did my residency and fellowship in neurology at Harvard, Peter Bent Brigham, and Beth Israel Children's Hospital in Boston.

Q. Where have you worked after you completed your training?

A. I was a staff neurologist at Harvard, initially as an instructor and subsequently as an Assistant Professor of neurology. Then I moved to Hawaii and have been a neurologist at Straub since 1975.

Q. Are you board-certified?

A. Yes. I'm board-certified by the American Board of Psychiatry and Neurology.

Q. Are you then also a psychiatrist?

A. Heavens, no!

(Comment: Some levity in a deposition is certainly appropriate and at times welcomed to ease an otherwise tense interchange. However, even an apparently innocent comment can backfire, as will be noted later in this deposition. See the last question on page 195.)

Q. Does your board certify both psychiatrists and neurologists?

A. That's correct.

Q. Do you belong to any medical societies or organizations?

A. I'm a member of the American Medical Association, the American Neurological Association, the American Association of Electrodiagnostic Medicine, and the Hawaii Medical Association.

Q. Now, Doctor, have you authored any articles in your field?

A. Yes.

Q. How many?

A. Nine.

Q. Have you ever testified in court before?

A. Yes.

Q. On how many occasions have you testified in court?

A. On more than 12 occasions.

Q. On each of those occasions, were you qualified as an expert witness in your specialty?

A. Yes.

Q. You practice in a specialized field of neurology, is that correct?

A. Yes.

Q. Could you explain what is encompassed in the field of neurology?

A. Neurology is the medical specialty that deals with disorders that affect the central nervous system, including the brain, brain stem and spinal cord, as well as the peripheral nervous system, including the peripheral nerves, muscles, and the neuromuscular junction.

Q. And you are testifying as an expert in neurology, is that correct?

A. Yes.

Attorney Asks How the Patient Was Referred

Q. In the course of your practice, are patients referred to you by other doctors or do they find you on their own?

A. Both.

Q. And in this case, how did Mr. Green come to see you?

A. He was referred by Dr. Gregory.

Q. How is Dr. Gregory known to you?

A. He's an internal medicine specialist at Straub.

Q. Here at the same facility?

A. Yes.

Q. You have with you your file on Mr. Green, don't you?

A. Yes.

Q. Could I see that, please?

A. Sure. This is his Straub chart, which includes his visits with me as well as other Straub doctors, and other test reports and correspondence related to his care.

Q. Could we have a copy of Mr. Green's Straub records attached as an exhibit to the deposition?

A. Yes, but could you do this through our Medical Records Department with the appropriate release forms signed?

Q. Of course. Can you make the arrangements with your Medical Records Department for us?

A. Sure.

Q. Doctor, when did you first see Mr. Green?

A. On October 5, 1994.

Q. What specifically were you asked to do?

A. I was asked by Dr. Gregory to provide a neurologic evaluation and offer an opinion and diagnosis of his headaches and various pain symptoms with respect to a motor vehicle accident of May 10, 1994.

Attorney Asks about the Evaluation

Q. And at the time that you first saw him, did you take a history from Mr. Green?

A. Yes.

Q. Could you relate to us what that was?

A. He told me that he was the driver of a car that was struck from behind by another automobile. His body went forward and his forehead struck the steering wheel. He said he lost consciousness briefly, and he immediately felt pain in his neck and lower back. He did not want any medical assistance from the ambulance attendants and was able to drive himself home, which is where he was headed. The next day he felt severe pain in his head and back areas and made an appointment to see his physician, Dr. Gregory. He said he could not remember some of the events of the day of the accident. He was treated by Dr. Gregory for about 5 months, but because of his persistent headaches and neck and back pain, the patient was referred to me for my opinion.

Q. And you conducted an examination, correct?

A. Yes.

Q. Were there any significant findings on examination?

A. Yes. His weight was 195 pounds, which was on the high side for somebody 5 feet 7½ inches tall. His pulse was 56, which is not in itself abnormal but indicative of a generally athletic person. The neck showed some mild spasm on far extension of movement. The neurologic examination showed a normal mental status as well as cranial nerve assessment. The sensory examination showed some decreased light touch sensation in the median distribution in both hands. Otherwise, the general neurologic examination produced normal findings.

Expert Explains Diagnoses

Q. Did you reach any diagnosis based on your evaluation of Mr. Green?

A. Yes. My diagnoses were cervical and lumbosacral strain, muscle contracture and posttraumatic headaches, and a mild closed-head injury, with concussion, from the accident. Also a diagnosis of bilateral carpal tunnel syndrome, which was not related to the accident of May 10, 1994.

Q. What does the term *strain* mean?

A. A strain would indicate that there is a muscle, ligament, or tendon type of injury and there is no neurologic injury, no nerve root problem, or a herniated disk.

Q. What is the physical mechanism of that type of injury?

A. Well, with the cervical strain, it could be a whipping motion, which laypeople term whiplash, or it could be a side-to-side movement, or it could be a torque or rotational type movement that is a forceful movement that causes strain on the neck.

Q. Can a cervical strain of the type you diagnosed also be caused by a direct trauma to the neck?

A. Yes.

Q. What do you mean by muscle contracture and posttraumatic headaches?

A. Muscle contracture relates to the tightening of neck muscles and the radiation of a pain to the scalp, which is interpreted as headache. Post-traumatic headaches can entail the same neck muscle mechanisms as well as indication of an injury that affects brain structures.

Q. Could you tell us what is meant by a closed head injury?

A. If you have an acute injury to the head region, it's a closed head injury when there is no fracture of the skull with exposed brain tissue, as opposed to an open head injury, when there's a fracture and exposure of brain tissue outside the confines of the skull.

Q. What do you mean by "with concussion"?

A. In Mr. Green's case, there was a head injury and a brief loss of consciousness. Also, he could not remember some of the things that preceded the accident and also after the accident. These facts would suggest that he suffered a mild concussion.

Q. In terms of the bilateral carpal tunnel syndrome, is it your opinion that that was not caused by the accident?

A. That's right. He had a pre-existing bilateral carpal tunnel syndrome since 1980.

Expert Describes Treatment

Q. Doctor, did you develop a plan of treatment for Mr. Green on that initial visit?

A. Yes. I went over my findings with him and I recommended that he should go for physical therapy.

Q. Tell us what happened.

A. He completed a series of physical therapy sessions and returned on October 30, 1994, stating he was better. He was taking occasional medications but not on a regular basis. His examination had shown no additional change and I suggested he continue to maintain therapy and see me in January 1995.

Q. For how long did he continue in physical therapy?

A. I gave him prescriptions until January 1995. However, he missed his January 22, 1995, and his February 28, 1995, visits with us. He did return, however, on May 8, 1995. He had stopped his physical therapy and why that happened I'm not sure. When I saw him in May he had some recurrence of his symptoms and noted that he was not having therapy at that time.

Q. Did he not show for the appointments in January and February?

A. Our records indicate that he didn't show for the January 22 appointment, but the February 28 appointment was rescheduled.

Q. Do you know why it was rescheduled?

A. No.

Q. In any event, when he came back to you in May, what was he complaining of?

A. He was still having musculoskeletal symptoms, which would be pain and aches. Also he had headaches, and therefore I suggested he try some additional medications. He also reported memory changes so I ordered neuropsychological testing.

Q. Did you tell him to continue with his physical therapy?

A. Yes. He continued physical therapy through May 30, 1995, and there's a note he canceled on June 4, 1995.

Q. Okay. What was the medication you put him on in May?

A. Inderal.

Q. What type of medication is that?

A. Inderal is a beta-blocker that's used for heart problems, blood pressure, and also migraine or vascular headaches, so I prescribed this to him. I also prescribed Esgic, which Dr. Gregory had given him for his headaches prior to his coming to see me. Esgic has a form of Tylenol called *acetaminophen*, also butalbital, which is a barbiturate, and caffeine.

Q. Is Esgic a pain medication?

A. Well, it's an analgesic, and more specifically beneficial for headache symptoms.

Q. Just briefly, what was your reason for referring him for neuropsychological testing?

A. First, to evaluate his memory problems, but also for opinions regarding any emotional factors that may be in play in this patient's symptoms.

Q. And what were the results of the neuropsychological testing?

A. Dr. Matthews, the neuropsychologist, found no organic brain injury, but did find evidence of a psychophysiological disorder, that is, a significant interplay between the patient's psychological state and his physical symptoms. Dr. Matthews recommended a trial of biofeedback sessions to treat the headaches and other pain symptoms, and I was in full agreement with those plans.

Q. What happened with the biofeedback sessions?

A. I saw Mr. Green on August 8, 1995, and at that time he reported doing better. He still had some neck and back pain and headaches. But he wanted to get back to work. In fact, he requested a work slip and I provided one to him.

Q. To be released by you medically?

A. Yes.

Attorney Questions Cause of Symptoms

Q. Do cervical and lumbosacral strains normally heal with time?

A. In a person who is 32, which he was at the time of the accident, strains normally heal physically within weeks, up to three months after the injury. This would happen in the large majority of persons who have no other disease. Now, if the person has a disease such as diabetes, forms of arthritis, or metabolic disease, then healing takes a longer period of time.

Q. In Mr. Green's case, did he have any history of disease?

A. No.

Q. So, at the time you last saw him in August 1995, well over a year after the accident, you expected the physical injuries to be healed, isn't that right?

A. Yes.

Q. So, as a neurologist, are you saying that when you last saw him, Mr. Green had no neurologic injury from the car accident?

A. Yes.

Q. If Mr. Green's physical injury from the car accident had healed, what was causing the symptoms he reported to you at your last examination?

A. It could be secondary to a systemic disease he had.

Q. Such as what?

A. He was on Esgic, a medication that could cause rebound pain when you don't take it. He had a previous history of back pain which wasn't completely resolved. There are other physical diseases that could be causing symptoms.

Q. So, am I to understand that, based on reasonable medical certainty, you don't have an opinion as to what was causing his symptoms at your last examination?

A. Whether they are neurologically or physically caused, that's correct. As far as a definitive cause, I don't think anyone could tell you that. The patient had a psychologist who treated him for his pain, so I would say a significant psychological factor plays a role here.

Q. But, heavens, you're no psychiatrist, are you? Can you really state that psychological factors are affecting the report of symptoms in this case?

A. By elimination of the fact that I find no neurologic cause, I feel that there are psychological factors, but I would defer to the psychologist as to the exact nature and relationship between the symptoms and the car accident of May 1994.

(Comment: A medical expert must be prepared to explain the causes of symptoms as clearly as possible. This witness gave a credible explanation for the patient's condition, albeit with some difficulty.)

Attorney Points Out Concussion Is Purely Patient's Report

Q. Now, with respect to your diagnosis of closed head injury with concussion, what importance did you place on the history that was given by the patient?

A. The history was very important.

Q. If in fact there was no loss of consciousness at the time of the accident, would that be of significance to you?

A. It's one aspect. There were other aspects in Mr. Green's case. He reported amnesia for events immediately before and after the accident. Also he told me about his forgetfulness since the head injury. That's why I ordered the neuropsychological examination.

Q. Which indicated no brain injury, right?

A. Yes.

Q. Now, the amnesia at the time of the accident, you could not determine that except for the history taken from the patient, is that correct?

A. Yes.

Q. Were you able to corroborate the report that Mr. Green was unconscious or had lost memory at the time of the accident?

A. No.

Q. Doctor, assume that at the time of the accident, Mr. Green was completely alert and could recall everything before and after the accident, would that affect your diagnosis?

Ms. Stevens: Note my objection to the hypothetical with facts not in evidence.

Mr. Vincent: Doctor, please answer the question.

A. Yes. My diagnosis would be closed-head injury without concussion.

(Comment: Many medical diagnoses are based on the patient's report. It is best to be able to provide corroborative evidence, such as witness's or family's observations. This witness's answers were direct, nondefensive, and honest.)

Attorney Raises Issue of Poor Motivation

Q. Now, referring to the physical therapy records and specifically with the notations of five cancellations and "poor motivation." Doctor, does that tell you something about Mr. Green and his complaints?

A. I don't know what you mean.

Q. Doesn't it tell you that he was not motivated to get better?

A. Well, it just says poor motivation for physical therapy because he had cancellations and no-shows.

Q. Okay, doesn't that indicate to you that he wasn't doing what he could have done in order to improve his condition?

A. That's hard to say. If he was having severe pain or headaches, that may have been his reason not to show. Or he might have had transportation problems or other conflicting obligations. Those would insinuate something very different.

Q. But the physical therapy record is something important that you take into account when you follow the patient during treatment, is it not?

A. Yes.

(Comment: It is wrong to defend poor treatment compliance, but it is equally wrong to make accusations without adequate facts. The witness did well not to simply agree with the physical therapist's inferences.)

A Pre-Existing Injury Is Noted

Q. Doctor, what is your understanding of Mr. Green's low back problem prior to the auto accident?

A. He had a work-related injury in 1988 involving a strain of his lower back.

Q. Do you have any idea of how symptomatic he was of low back problems up until the 1994 auto accident?

A. He said he was about 75% better from the previous injury and not back to normal. However, he was able to work full-time as a sales representative for auto parts.

Q. Okay. So was his condition stable at that time?

A. That's hard to say. I believe it was stable.

Q. Didn't you obtain a computed tomographic scan of his lower back?

A. I did.

Q. Do you recall your conclusions regarding the CT scan?

A. The radiologist concluded that there were degenerative changes but there was no herniated disk.

Q. Degenerative changes mean changes that occur over a long period of time as opposed to, say, a traumatic type injury?

A. No, I don't think you could say that. You could get degenerative changes from within 6 months or so.

Q. Did you see any differences between the CT scans that were taken before, compared with the CT scan taken after the auto accident?

A. I didn't have the opportunity to look at the scan that was taken at the time of the work injury.

Q. Did you see the reports of the CT scans?

A. Yes, I did.

Q. And what comparisons were you able to make between the two injuries?

A. You can say the auto accident did not worsen his anatomical presentation, based on those reports.

Q. In your report you indicated some findings of a bulging disk that you concluded as a result of your neurological examination. Did that pre-exist the auto accident?

A. I believe so.

(Comment: The attorney has carefully and craftily elicited evidence of a pre-existing low back problem. The witness responded accurately to the inquiry and avoided advocating for the patient or his lawyer.)

Witness Is Asked to Apportion Injuries

Q. Going back to the cervical and lumbosacral strain, did you reach any opinions as to apportionment on that?

A. I haven't been asked to do that.

Q. Did you feel that his injuries were solely caused by the May 10, 1994, accident, or you just don't know?

A. The May 10, 1994, accident versus the 1988 work injury?

Q. Yes. The 1988 injury as well as anything else that may have pre-existed.

Ms. Stevens: Objection. I don't know if the doctor has a proper foundation to answer that question because I don't know to what extent he reviewed the records of the 1988 work injury. But, Doctor, you can try to answer.

A. Mr. Green had low back problems from the work injury of 1988. He had symptoms that did not completely resolve by the time of the 1994 car accident, but he had been able to work full-time without medical care for over three years. In my opinion, with regard to the symptoms that remain, I would estimate that about 80% are due to the car accident and the remainder to the previous work injury as they relate to the musculoskeletal soft tissue symptoms of his neck and back.

(Comment: If there is insufficient information, the expert witness should not attempt to apportion the effects of the two injuries. When no apportionment is made by the expert, the jury will probably assume the responsibility of apportioning the plaintiff's medical problems.)

Witness Is Asked for a Prognosis

Q. Did you have a prognosis as to recovery or physical healing in terms of the cervical and lumbosacral strain?

A. Well, at the time I first saw him in October 1994, I couldn't give you a prognosis. Subsequently, when I saw him and his symptoms were less, the prognosis was that there would be healing of the strain. But that's not addressing the issue of symptoms, which are subjective.

Q. As of the last time you saw the patient on August 8, 1995, did you have a prognosis?

A. The prognosis for the physical healing of the soft tissue injury to his neck and back was that it would heal or had healed. Whether he would have symptoms I couldn't answer at that point.

Q. I take it then, it's your opinion with regard to the symptomatology that you cannot say how long that would continue as of August 8, 1995?

A. That's correct.

Q. But from a physical standpoint, the injuries would heal in a short time thereafter?

A. Yes, but for some people that period of time is not so short. It may be short for some people but not for others.

Q. Doctor, if the patient has neck and back pain today, would you say that these symptoms are related to the accident of May 10, 1994?

A. The neck and back pain he had when I saw him was related to the May 10, 1994, accident, but whether that accident accounts for his present symptoms, over 2 years later, I can't say because there is no repeat CT scan to see if his back has gotten worse or not.

Q. And with regard to the closed-head injury, did you have a prognosis as of the last time you saw him?

A. Yes.

Q. What was the prognosis?

A. The prognosis was good. He had no neurologic residual and would have full recovery of that.

(Comment: In medicolegal cases a prognosis is critical in determining the appropriate compensatory award. Sometimes physicians can confidently provide a prognosis; at other times they simply do not have a crystal ball. This witness did his best to be truthful and accurate.)

Attorney Asks about Future Evaluations

Q. Do you have any scheduled appointments to see Mr. Green in the near future?

A. No.

Q. Do you have any plans to re-evaluate him?

A. No.

Q. And I take it you haven't been asked to see him again in the near future?

A. That's right.

Q. If you do see Mr. Green again, could someone let my office know about this?

Ms. Stevens: We certainly would do that.
Mr. Vincent: I have no further questions. Thank you.
Ms. Stevens: I have a few.

Plaintiff Attorney Cross-Examines

Q. Doctor, you've treated hundreds, even thousands of patients who have been in auto accidents, correct?

A. Yes.

Q. Some people get in automobile accidents and recover quickly, some never recover, and some in between, obviously, right?

A. Yes.

Q. And you've treated all of those kinds of patients, correct?

A. Yes.

Q. The symptoms that Mr. Green presents with, Doctor, are those in any way out of the ordinary for a low-speed impact between two cars?

A. No.

Ms. Stevens: I have no further questions.

Closing Arguments

The sample deposition in this chapter typifies the kind of questioning that takes place in a pretrial oral deposition of a treating physician. The deposition covered basic information about the witness's qualifications, how the patient was referred to the doctor, the examinations, and the treatments. The deposing attorney asked challenging questions pertaining to etiology, the patient's subjective reports, motivational issues, and a pre-existing condition. The expert witness was also asked to apportion the injuries since there was apparently more than one contributing factor, that is, a previous injury.

The physician in this deposition offered his opinions in a straightforward professional manner. He provided honest and accurate answers, whether or not they assisted his patient's case, and avoided being his patient's advocate. He acknowledged having limited information in certain areas, such as corroborative evidence for the patient's alleged loss of consciousness and amnesia. He remained within the scope of his expertise as a neurologist and appropriately deferred to the opinion of the psychologist with respect to specific psychological issues of the case. While he expressed certitude in many instances, he was also willing to say "I don't know" when that was the best answer.

The physician witness in this case demonstrated the benefits of his years of experience in medicolegal cases. Note that he kept his answers short and to the point, not volunteering unnecessary information and yet being responsive to each question asked. What he was able to do in his deposition is not beyond the scope of the reader who becomes familiar with the ground rules of expert testifying, the adversarial nature of legal proceedings, and the various strategies and tactics of the deposing attorney.

11

Final Closing Arguments

In clinical practice, the medical doctor labors as a humanitarian and healer in roles that are honored in all sectors of our community. In the courtroom, the medical doctor functions principally as a scientific educator, and although the task of an expert witness may not be as inspiring or satisfying as that of a health care professional, the role of the physician testifying in court shares equal importance in our civilized society. The physician witness who testifies at a criminal trial, in a personal injury lawsuit, in a medical malpractice case, or at an administrative hearing for disability benefits fulfills a critical obligation to the community because the jurisprudence system requires medical expertise to resolve many of its disputes.

The physician witness has not always succeeded in contributing to legal justice. The unprepared witness, the physician who offers junk science testimony, the physician who testifies outside the scope of his or her expertise, the polished professional witness who sways jurors on the basis of rhetoric or emotions, and the ignominious "hired gun" serve no useful purpose in the courtroom. These physicians do great harm to themselves and the medical profession, but, more seriously, they fail to safeguard the rights and freedoms of individuals involved in the legal process.

In spite of the fact that medicine, as a science, has its fallibilities, medical doctors are being summoned by the legal profession with increasing frequency for a variety of criminal and civil proceedings. The litigious atmosphere of today's society is reflected in the explosion of lawsuits in America as well as other Western societies, such as Great

Britain, Canada, and Australia, and the courts believe that a physician's expertise is a sine qua non to unravel the complexities of its many medicolegal disputes.

To be an effective medical witness, it is clearly not enough to have merely completed medical school or to have the esteemed board credentials. The physician must have not only a firm grasp of updated medical knowledge in his or her specialty but also must understand the basic tenets of law, its interface with medicine, and especially the adversarial nature in its search for truth and justice. The duty of the physician witness is to formulate medical opinions based on solid objective evidence and to communicate these findings in a clear and persuasive manner to the triers of fact so that they can reach a fair and just determination of the case. To be credible, the physician witness must be able to defend his or her testimony against skillful oppositional challenges and to remain the calm, confident, and impartial professional.

How does a physician obtain the knowledge and skill required to be an effective medical expert witness? Organized medicine offers criteria to qualify medical experts and provides basic ethical guidelines but leaves many questions about the interface of medicine and the law unanswered. Having no training or courtroom experience, the uninformed medical witness will find testifying to be, at best, anxiety-provoking and unpleasant or, at worst, a professional disaster for the physician and a shameful example for the profession as a whole. Gee and Mason, both professors of forensic medicine in Great Britain, have recommended that all doctors be trained for the role as medical expert witnesses during their medical school or residency training,[1] but there are few, if any, such instructional programs for physicians.[1] Some have suggested that residency programs routinely review medical malpractice cases and the associated testimony by physician witnesses. This case review process would introduce residents to the legal realities of medical practice, provide a forum to critique medical testimony, and teach residents how to interact with the legal system.[2]

Several professional societies and individuals have now organized workshops and produced textbooks for expert witness testifying. While these educational efforts are beneficial to many, Jones warns that the advice often appears to emphasize how to help a legal case rather than to help the medical witness.[3] With limited learning opportunities available, most physicians have had to rely on on-the-job training.[4] Indeed, the more experience physicians have in courtroom testifying, the better their understanding of the medicolegal system and the more likely they can cope with the complex task of a medical expert. Furthermore, physician witnesses should not testify in secrecy but should be encouraged to share their depositions and seek peer review of their sworn testimony. More open discussion, such as at grand rounds, can improve the quality of expert testifying and encourage more qualified physicians to participate as expert witnesses.[5]

This book was written to provide a basic understanding of the role of the physician in the legal system, with detailed approaches on how effective testimony can be offered. It would behoove you to review the poorly thought-out answers in this book and practice the calmer style of responding, especially those readers who are prone to high anxiety and impulsive retorts in the face of grueling questioning. Although some physicians have a natural ability in public speaking and excel in court, we believe that when properly prepared almost everyone can be a good witness. With sufficient skills for testifying in court and coping with aggressive cross-examination, the medical witness will succeed in assisting the court in important medicolegal matters.

There may be concern by some that the suggestions in the foregoing chapters will simply train physicians to become polished expert witnesses who can successfully manipulate the triers of fact. It may be unavoidable that certain unscrupulous individuals, who want to profit from a potentially lucrative career of courtroom testifying, may capitalize from the many tips in this book. However, this is clearly not the purpose of the book.

Physicians who are called on to testify should be concerned with truth and justice, and the responsibility of determining what the truth is and what justice is rests with the individual physician. Throughout this book we have urged physicians to accept the responsibility of testifying in court, to support their testimony with firm scientific evidence, to acknowledge the limits of the evidence as well as their expertise, and to remain objective and impartial medical witnesses. When these principles are upheld, physicians provide an invaluable service to our system of jurisprudence.

See you in court.

References

1. Gee DJ, Mason JK. *The Courts and the Doctor.* Oxford, England: Oxford University Press, 1990.
2. Fish R, Ehrhardt M. Review of medical negligence cases: an essential part of residency programs. *J Emerg Med* 1992;10:501–504.

3. Jones CAG. *Expert Witnesses: Science, Medicine and the Practice of Law.* Oxford, England: Clarendon Press, 1994.
4. Nicholson JL. Expert testimony for the defense: learning from practical experience. *Forensic Examiner* 1997;6:20–24.
5. Brent RL. The irresponsible medical witness: a failure of biomedical graduate education and professional accountability. *Pediatrics* 1982;70:754–762.

Federal Rules of Evidence

The Federal Rules of Evidence are liberal with respect to the admissibility of expert opinions and the discretion they confer on trial judges.

- Testimony by experts: Rule 702 authorizes judges to admit expert scientific or medical testimony if it "will assist the trier of fact to understand the evidence or to determine a fact in issue." To testify under this federal rule, an expert must qualify "by knowledge, skill, experience, training, or education." As it is written, this language affords courts broad latitude in determining what testimony it will hear and from whom.

- Bases of opinion testimony by experts: Rule 703 allows an expert to base an opinion on data "perceived by or made known to him at or before the hearing." The information relied on need not be admissible into evidence if "of a type reasonably relied upon by experts in the particular field in forming opinions or inferences on the subject." Hence, a medical expert can base an opinion not only on his or her personal evaluation of a patient but also on reports of others' examinations or on a review of records, whether or not these data are themselves admissible as evidence.

- Disclosure of facts or data underlying expert opinion: Rule 705 allows an expert to offer an opinion "without proper disclosure of the underlying facts or data, unless the court requires otherwise." However, this does not shield the expert from having to "disclose the underlying facts or data on cross-examination." This federal rule is partly designed to expedite trials by allowing experts to testify before the data on which they rely are admitted as evidence.

Expansive as these federal rules may be, they yet empower trial courts to exclude or limit expert testimony they perceived as flawed.

- Excluding expert testimony: Rule 402 permits courts to exclude otherwise relevant expert testimony if "its probative value is substantially outweighed by danger of unfair prejudice, confusion of the issues, or misleading the jury." Hence, if opposing counsel can convince a court that an expert's opinion is biased or likely to mislead a jury, the court can exclude it.

- Court-appointed experts: Rule 706 permits trial judges to appoint their own expert witnesses if they so choose. Therefore, if judges find scientific evidence difficult to understand or evaluate or they are uncomfortable about the reliability of proffered expert testimony from partisan witnesses, they can select neutral experts to assist them in determining what testimony should be admitted.

In spite of these residual judicial powers to exclude flawed testimony, many attorneys, judges, and legal commentators have opined that too much "junk science" is presented before trial courts and that remedial steps are in order.

- *Daubert v. Merrell Dow Pharmaceuticals*, 125 SCt 469 (1993): This case may be the first important step. The Supreme Court's opinion strongly signals to trial courts that they should exercise initiative in weighing offers of scientific testimony. No longer will it suffice to merely determine relevance; courts must also address the issue of reliability, even if this requires preliminary hearings of extensive types. Now some federal trial courts are holding "Daubert hearings" and proffered testimony of "hired guns" is attracting increasing scrutiny.

B

Annotated Reference List

Appelbaum PS, Gutheil TG (eds). *Clinical Handbook of Psychiatry and the Law* (2nd ed). Baltimore: Williams & Wilkins, 1991.

The second edition of this award-winning text gives psychiatrists a practical and accessible guide to the relationship between psychiatry and the complexities of the legal world. Issues such as patient rights, confidentiality, negligent supervision, acquired immunodeficiency syndrome, and increasing health care costs are addressed in light of the rapid growth of malpractice suits facing mental health professionals.

Babitsky S, Mangraviti JJ Jr. *How to Excel During Cross-Examination: Techniques for Experts that Work*. Falmouth, MA: SEAK, 1997.

Written by two attorneys, this book is designed to be a comprehensive yet easy-to-use guide for expert witnesses preparing for cross-examination. Included are sample cross-examinations from leading experts and attorneys from across the United States. By understanding the types of questions that may be asked, the expert witness can learn to excel during cross-examination.

Horsley JE. *Testifying in Court: A Guide for Physicians* (4th ed). Los Angeles: Product Information Management, 1992.

This book is a basic manual for the physician who needs to know what is involved when called to testify in court. The author emphasizes how to prepare for testifying, how to determine proper fees, and most importantly, how to be an effective witness.

James AE Jr (ed). *Legal Medicine: With Special Reference to Diagnostic Imaging.* Baltimore: Urban & Schwarzenberg, 1980.

Written by recognized authorities in medicine and law, this text presents a wide range of pertinent subjects including the elements of malpractice trials, cross-examination, diagnostic specialists as expert witnesses, forensic radiology, and defensive medicine. The volume familiarizes physicians with the courtroom experience and provides attorneys with a greater comprehension of the medical system vis-à-vis litigation.

Liebenson HA. *You, the Expert Witness.* Mundelein, IL: Callaghan & Company, 1962.

This book, written by an attorney in 1962, remains a useful handbook for physicians and other professionals who are called into court by the attorney of a party in a lawsuit. The objective of the book is to introduce the language and procedures of the courtroom, which will enable the reader to be more at ease while on the witness stand.

Matson JV. *Effective Expert Witnessing: A Handbook for Technical Professionals.* Chelsea, MI: Lewis Publishers, 1990.

Written for technical professionals, this handbook on expert witnessing discusses the battles that characterize legal war in a courtroom. The reader will become familiar with the mind games employed and learn ways to fight the intellectual battles with knowledge of the strategies that are used in trials when technology and law intersect. The author is an engineering professor and a lawyer.

Rossi FF (ed). *Expert Witnesses.* Chicago: American Bar Association, 1991.

Published by the American Bar Association, this text is written for the trial lawyer who today needs a solid grasp of the law regulating expert witnesses and of the practical techniques for managing their testimony. Prominent trial attorneys contribute chapters devoted to the handling of experts in specific fields, such as medicine and psychiatry.

Tsushima WT, Anderson RM Jr. *Mastering Expert Testimony: A Courtroom Handbook for Mental Health Professionals.* Mahwah, NJ: Lawrence Erlbaum, 1996.

This book emphasizes the typical courtroom dialogue between attorneys and mental health professionals who are testifying about their psychotherapy patients or who are hired by lawyers specifically to provide expert opinions. The book is based on the belief that exposure to courtroom dialogue enhances the awareness of appropriate professional responses to an attorney's cross-examination and greatly alleviates the fears about a situation that is known to provoke intense levels of anxiety.

Vevaina JR, Bone RC, Kassoff E (eds). *Legals Aspects of Medicine: Including Cardiology, Pulmonary Medicine, and Critical Care Medicine.* New York: Springer-Verlag, 1989.

This is a book written by experts in law and medicine. New government laws and regulations have had a deep impact on medicine, and biomedical technology and research have created new legal questions that have not been considered before. This book will be of interest to those who work in the fields of law and medicine, particularly those who specialize in cardiology, pulmonology, and critical care medicine.

Zobel HB, Rous SR. *Doctors and the Law.* New York: WW Norton, 1993.

Coauthored by a judge and a physician, this book offers help to the physician who is facing a malpractice lawsuit. The book is aimed at helping the distressed physician cope with a new and traumatic experience as a defendant as well as a witness.

C

Expert Witness Checklist

Pretrial Preparation

1. Understand the medical expertise required for the case.
2. Determine what pretrial work is requested.
3. Clarify the fee arrangements.
4. Review thoroughly the file and relevant information.
5. Understand the medical issues in the case.
6. Determine the strengths and weaknesses of your testimony.
7. Cooperate with court-ordered subpoenas.
8. Prepare a current curriculum vitae.
9. Meet with the attorney to discuss your testimony.
10. Prepare to take to court what the subpoena requires.

Presentation in Court

1. Dress professionally.
2. Arrive at the courthouse before your scheduled appearance.
3. Sit erect and avoid nervous gestures.

4. Pay attention to each question.

5. Speak firmly with a strong voice.

6. Use everyday language.

7. Present objective testimony based on sound medical reasoning.

8. Answer precisely only what is asked.

9. Stay within your area of expertise.

10. Avoid advocating for one side.

D

Primer on Medical Malpractice

Many physicians will be sued for medical malpractice during the course of their professional careers. In preparing for that eventuality, physicians should practice the most meticulous medicine to avoid lawsuits and be optimally defensible in a court of law.

What Is Malpractice?

Malpractice pertains to professional negligence, and it applies to physicians, attorneys, engineers, and other professionals who function improperly in the performance of duties, whether intentionally or through carelessness or ignorance. Malpractice denotes the negligent or unskillful performance of duties during a person's professional relationship with patients or clients.

What Constitutes a Medical Malpractice Claim?

1. The physician had a duty to care for the plaintiff.

2. The physician failed in the duty to care.

3. The failure to provide appropriate care was a proximate cause of the plaintiff's injury.

4. The injury can be measured for compensation in monetary damages.

When Is a Physician Negligent in the Duty to Care?

• When the physician departs from commonly accepted standards of medical practice

• When the physician fails to keep abreast of changes in medical practice

• When the physician uses a new but unproven and unaccepted method of treatment

• When the physician fails to take precautions against risks

• When the physician does not perform to the standards of his or her specialty

Reasons for Medical Malpractice Lawsuits

• Poor medical results

• Unreasonable patient expectations

• Inaccurate predictions by physician

• Unexpected complications

• Litigious society

Potential Medicolegal Problems

• Failure to admit to hospital

• Delay in diagnosis

• Erroneous diagnosis

• Failure or delay in performing procedure

Diagnostic Procedures That Can Result in Malpractice Claims

• Angiography

• Procedures using contrast medium

- Venipuncture
- Lumbar puncture
- Electromyography and nerve conduction studies
- Other invasive procedures

Medications That Can Result in Malpractice Claims

- Birth control pills
- Anticoagulants
- Tetracycline
- Theophylline
- Anticonvulsants
- Long-term steroid therapy
- Demerol in head trauma cases
- Chemotherapy
- Radiotherapy

Laboratory Activity That Can Result in Malpractice Claims

- Failure to perform requested test
- Delayed reports

Hospital/Staff Interactions That Can Result in Malpractice Claims

- Failure to transfer
- Diet inappropriate for medical condition
- Housekeeping orders (e.g., neglecting sterilization requirements)
- Visitation that affects patient's health

E

Algorithms for Expert Testifying*

These flow charts may assist in your decisions pertaining to medical testifying.

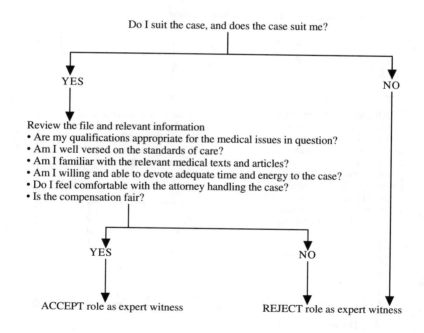

Do I suit the case, and does the case suit me?

YES → Review the file and relevant information
• Are my qualifications appropriate for the medical issues in question?
• Am I well versed on the standards of care?
• Am I familiar with the relevant medical texts and articles?
• Am I willing and able to devote adequate time and energy to the case?
• Do I feel comfortable with the attorney handling the case?
• Is the compensation fair?

NO

YES → ACCEPT role as expert witness

NO → REJECT role as expert witness

REJECT role as expert witness

---

*The algorithms on pages 220 and 221 are modifications of graphical explanations prepared by David L. Faigman, law professor at the Hastings College of Law of the University of California.

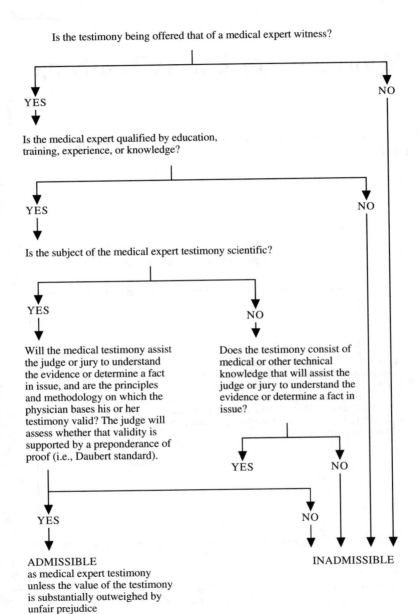

Is the testimony being offered that of a medical expert witness?

YES   **NO**

Is the medical expert qualified by education, training, experience, or knowledge?

YES   **NO**

Is the subject of the medical expert testimony scientific?

YES   **NO**

Will the medical testimony assist the judge or jury to understand the evidence or determine a fact in issue, and are the principles and methodology on which the physician bases his or her testimony valid? The judge will assess whether that validity is supported by a preponderance of proof (i.e., Daubert standard).

Does the testimony consist of medical or other technical knowledge that will assist the judge or jury to understand the evidence or determine a fact in issue?

YES   **NO**

YES   **NO**

ADMISSIBLE
as medical expert testimony unless the value of the testimony is substantially outweighed by unfair prejudice

INADMISSIBLE

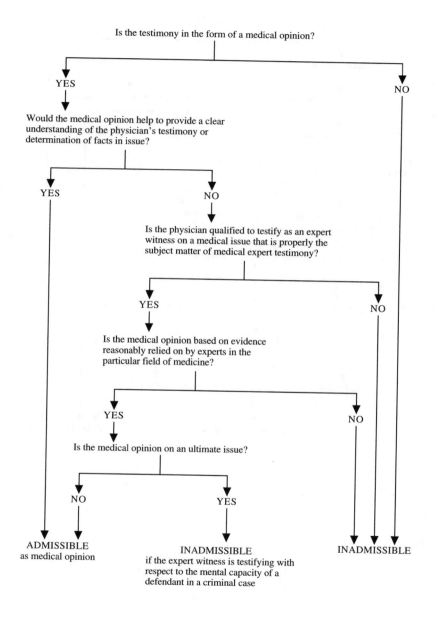

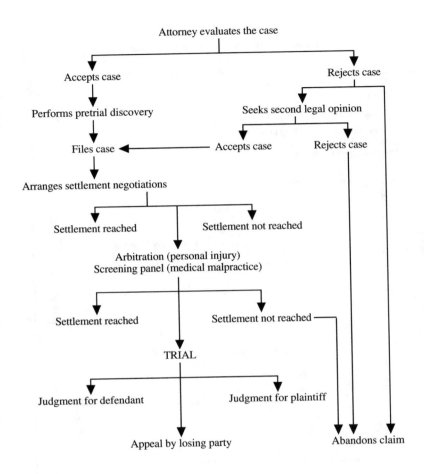

Index